Praise for *Solving the Autoimmune Puzzle*

"*Solving the Autoimmune Puzzle* is functional medicine at its best. Dr. Keesha Ewers integrates her wealth of knowledge from behavioral science, Ayurvedic medicine, and functional medicine to create an easy to use system that gets to the core of real healing. This book is full of practical information and tools that will free all who use it from pain and suffering of any kind, including autoimmune disease."

—**Dr. Mark Hyman**, New York Times bestselling author of *Eat Fat, Get Thin*. Director, *Cleveland Clinic Center for Functional Medicine*.

"I applaud Dr. Ewers for bringing to light two very often overlooked root causes for those suffering with autoimmunity: stress and trauma. In her book, *Solving the Autoimmune Puzzle: The Woman's Guide to Reclaiming Emotional Freedom and Vibrant Health*, Dr. Ewers dives deep into emotional aspects of those with autoimmunity and shows the reader how to come to peace with themselves and their trauma allowing them to heal from autoimmunity."

—**Amy Myers, MD**, New York Times bestselling author of *The Autoimmune Solution* and *The Thyroid Connection*.

"Dr. Keesha Ewers lays out a clear, easy-to-follow roadmap to break free from inflammation and autoimmune disease. Her insightful, well-researched plan uncovers the missing pieces of the autoimmune puzzle and shows how to reverse this century's greatest health challenge for women."

—**JJ Virgin, CNS, CHFS**, NYT bestselling author of *The Virgin Diet & Sugar Impact Diet*

"*Solving the Autoimmune Puzzle* provides you with a straight forward way to understand the root causes of complex diseases of all kinds, including autoimmunity. Dr. Keesha Ewers shares ways to reverse autoimmune disease in a way that is doable, and she does it using humor, wisdom, and science. This is a must read for all women and for all who love women."

—**Dr. Christine Horner**, author of *Waking the Warrior Goddess*

"Dr. Keesha Ewers' book contains information about the key factors involved in the cause and cure of autoimmune diseases. She can be your life coach and help you to terminate the self-destructive nature of this disease, I have seen the benefit of her wisdom in patients when they learn how to let love and forgiveness into their lives and free them from their prison and disease."

—**Bernie Siegel, MD**, author of *365 Prescriptions for the Soul* and *A Book of Miracles*

"*Solving the Autoimmune Puzzle* brings together the best of Western medicine, Ayurveda, functional medicine, and clinical practice into an accessible and exciting system for taking charge of your health, life, and happiness. Dr. Keesha Ewers has applied her knowledge, humor, and clinical wisdom to create a healing masterpiece that will benefit any reader. Highly recommended!"

—**Dr. Keith Witt**, author of *Integral Mindfulness: From Clueless to Dialed-in*, and *Shadow Light: Illuminations at the Edge of Darkness.*

"Dr. Keesha Ewers is a Renaissance woman for the 21st century. Trained in cutting-edge medical science, she is also attuned to the subtleties of nature, the nuances of energy flow, and the healing power of spiritual truths from a variety of disciplines. All of these make *Solving the Autoimmune Puzzle* an innovative, comprehensive guide to help us become more aware of our uniqueness—with scores of practical ways to care for ourselves: body, mind, heart, and spirit."

—**Gina Ogden, PhD, LMFT**, bestselling and award-winning author of *Expanding the Practice of Sex Therapy, The Return of Desire,* and other books.

"This is a Magnum Opus! *Solving the Autoimmune Puzzle* is an encyclopedic accomplishment with flair! Dr. Ewers has elucidated the strengths of Western medicine and the weaknesses with complete lucidity. My head was spinning with admiration at the formatting and expositions of this material. May this book benefit all."

—**Dr. Jonn Mumford (Swami Anandakapila Saraswati)**, author of *Psychosomatic Yoga, Ecstasy Through Tantra* and *A Chakra and Kundalini Workbook.*

"Dr. Keesha Ewers delivers a penetrating diagnosis of an ailment that afflicts tens of millions of people—and she offers a powerful holistic prescription. You'll find wisdom for your body, mind, heart and spirit—and support to help you bring your hormones, neurology, and life into balance."

—**Ocean Robbins, CEO**, The Food Revolution Network.

"With true compassion, a sense of humor, and wise honesty Dr Keesha Ewers combines her personal journey of physical, emotional and spiritual transformation with her professional functional medicine background to outline a clear, easy-to-implement Self Help path to address all underlying root causes of the various expressions of autoimmune disease. She takes the reader by the hand and offers evidence-based guidance and practical steps that leave the conventional medical paradigm in the dust to offer true and lasting solutions to the many chronic health problems plaguing millions of women in today's sophisticated world. This is a MUST read for anyone wishing to embark on a holistic healing path."

—**Kirstin Nussgruber, CNC, EMB**, author of *Confessions of a Cancer Conqueror. My 5 Step Process to Transform Your Relationship with Cancer.*

"Dr. Ewers' insightful exploration of autoimmunity brings to the discussion two incredibly important components—the role of traumatic experiences and chronic stress. With humor and honesty, she shares her own journey of pain, illness and ultimate recovery, as she elucidates the wisdom of traditional medicine coupled with the findings of modern bio-medicine, to bring forth a roadmap of recouping one's health to attain true vitality. A profound, engaging read for anyone struggling with any kind of autoimmune presentation—*Solving the Autoimmune Puzzle: The Woman's Guide to Reclaiming Emotional Freedom and Vibrant Health* will educate and inspire a very different view of the road to illness and the healing from it."

—**Sarica Cernohous, LAc., MSTOM, BSBA**, author of *The Funky Kitchen: Easy Techniques from Our Ancestors for Improved Digestion, Enhanced Vitality and Joy!*

SOLVING THE
AUTOIMMUNE
PUZZLE

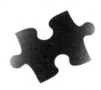

The Woman's Guide to Reclaiming
Emotional Freedom and Vibrant Health

Dr. Keesha Ewers

samadhi
press

First Printing: 2017

Printed in USA

Samadhi Press

Library of Congress Control Number: 2017938275

Book Design by Adele Wiejaczka

DR. KEESHA EWERS

4410 Newport Way NW

Issaquah, WA USA 98027

(425) 391–3376

info@DrKeesha.com

www.DrKeesha.com

ORDERING INFORMATION

Special discounts are available on quantity purchases by corporations, associations, educators, and others. For details, contact the publisher at the above listed address.

BOOKING, PRESS & SPEAKING INQUIRIES

www.DrKeesha.com/contact

"The world will be saved by the Western woman."

"If we are going to see real development in the world, then our best investment is in women."

DEDICATION

For my patients and students: I am continually touched and inspired with your courage and wisdom.

For my children: powerful, gentle, courageous, and constantly evolving in the most amazing ways.

For my parents: Thank you for laying the groundwork, for life, and for being such amazing examples.

For my beloved: You are my mirror and my sandpaper. Thank you for your devotion and willingness.

For Ramana Maharshi: Eternal gratitude for opening the doorway between the worlds.

CONTENTS

FOREWORD BY DR. TOM O'BRYAN

A question: Do you remember meeting someone in your life and just felt good from meeting them? Just being with them and you felt 'lit up', a bit happier-just as a result of meeting them? My experience is those people you meet who light you up are the 'treasures' of humanity. They've found something inside of them that just naturally radiates, is contagious, and most of us want more of that.

On the other hand, most people are 'surviving' in life. When you see someone you know and you say "Hi. How are you", how often do you hear "fine, how are you", or "not bad", or some other quick, deflective answer. Many of you have heard my interpretation in the past of the response, 'fine', to mean 'feeling insecure, neurotic, and emotional'.

You don't need to work with your 'emotional self' very much to survive in this world. But if you want to be a torch to others, or if you want to attract more of the people in your life who light you up, reading Dr. Keesha Ewer's book is a roadmap to more inner peace that will let your inner light shine.

For many, in the long list of causality of autoimmune disease, a commonly overlooked, yet impactful part of the puzzle is early childhood trauma. To leave this avenue of recovery orphaned and unattended is to leave true healing beyond our reach, and that is a tragedy. Dr. Keesha Ewers has pulled the curtain back on the ACE (Adverse Childhood Experiences) study and invited all of us to look closely and fearlessly at the phantom hiding under the bed. Only in that space do you find a critical contributor to the dis-ease you may be suffering from.

Dr. Keesha has devoted her life to not only uncovering the healing but to carrying it to the world at large through her work as a practitioner and now as an author.

Through my decades of study on the impact of gluten and the connection to autoimmunity, I know the deep drive to be an ambassador into the puzzle that others simply navigate around. That courage, to look into the ACE score and find the missing piece of the puzzle is a mirror for me to my own work over these decades with wheat related disorders and autoimmune disease.

Autoimmune disorders now cumulatively make up the third leading cause of death in the industrialized world. Recognized in about 50 million people, but only 1 out of 3 are diagnosed, diagnosable autoimmunity is present in at least 72 million people in the US.

To provide a context to evaluate the impact of autoimmune diseases, cancer affected approximately 9 million people and heart disease affected approximately 22 million people in the United States.

We know that you are 10 times more likely to develop an autoimmune disorder if you have celiac disease. How far early childhood trauma goes into those cases and would provide an avenue for healing is the great frontier.

You might say...I am on a mission. And so is Dr. Keesha Ewers.

I can almost guarantee that your doctor, gastroenterologist or even your specialist doesn't know much of this information on ACE scores and probably doesn't grasp its potential significance.

For many, the lifelong impact of unresolved trauma lies dormant and unrecognized—and unhealed—unless pioneers like Dr. Keesha fearlessly shine a light on.

We are only beginning to understand the impact of stress on health and Health Care Practitioners are working to bring healing modalities into that space. The observation Dr. Keesha makes in this book is that no child is without trauma, it is a matter of degree. We must bring healing modalities into this in the same way we are attempting to at least recognize stress as a contributing factor to health in our present lives.

In this book, adverse childhood experiences are defined and measured in a way the reader can understand, identify within themselves and begin to create a healing protocol that will help change the understanding and impact of autoimmunity forever.

This is a large missing piece of the puzzle to "why do I have____ (whatever the dis-ease is that you are suffering with). We are down to where the roots of disease live. Successful use of medication addresses symptoms-that's what drugs do (and 'Thank God' they work as often as they do). But without addressing the hidden triggers causing the imbalance, the triggers will just manifest somewhere else in the body.

Once again, you don't need to work with your 'emotional self' very much to survive in this world. Life can be 'fine' without looking in these corners of your mind. But to be one of those who 'light up' your children, or your family, or the world, and to address the underlying triggers to whatever dis-ease you are suffering from, this book is an essential piece of the puzzle.

~DR. TOM O'BRYAN

ACKNOWLEDGEMENTS

I must begin by acknowledging the women who have gone before me. The freedom I have to live my life path is because of all that you did before I was even born. My deepest thanks to my teachers and mentors, without whom I would still be stuck in an upset 10-year-old's belief system.

Many thanks to Madge Warner and Bishop Rasmussen, who reached out and loved a young woman who was a firebrand. Thank you to the first mentor I intentionally sought out to emulate in parenting and aging with grace, Bonnie Wright. Your friendship and wisdom are still today appreciated deeply.

Thank you to Swami Rama for bringing me through to my "next level" of development and blowing the limitations open of what I thought was possible. My deepest appreciation to the Seattle interfaith community, Becky Bell, Walter Andrews and the East Shore parents for your support of the most amazing group of young people I had the blessing and honor of helping to shepherd through adolescence.

Thank you to Dr. Helen Palmer, Diane Zimberhoff, Dr. David Grand, Dr. Vasant Lad, Dr. Vivek Shanbhag, the teachers at the *Institute for Functional Medicine*, and Dr. Gina Ogden for your mentorship. Being a part of the Mindshare community is priceless and something I am grateful for each and every day.

Thank you to my team, both online and at *Fern Life Center*, what an incredible group of people I have the honor and blessing to work with! Nicky and Mary Agnes, your devotion to this work has made it come to fruition. And of course, my patients at *Fern Life Center* and students in the *Academy for Integrative Medicine* health coach certification program are the reason I keep up-leveling my practice. What an incredible group of human beings!

Sweet appreciation to my medicine teachers Mother Aya, Puma and Apu Huachuma. My eternal thanks to my Tantric teacher, Swami Anandakapila Saraswati, for his spiritual guidance and teachings as this project was created. My children light up my life and are my constant source of joy. And finally, I want to express just how grateful I am to my husband for his constant love, support and editorial assistance in bringing this book to life. And to the *Absolute, Arunachala, the Hill of Wisdom*, whose fire burns ever in my heart, shining the way for this mystic to express her dharma into the world.

INTRODUCTION

"Healing does not mean going back to the way things were before, but rather allowing what is now to move us closer to God."

~**RAM DASS**

Women are diagnosed with 80% of the over 145 identified autoimmune diseases (that number is still growing). Several autoimmune diseases, including lupus, rheumatoid arthritis, Hashimoto's thyroiditis, myasthenia gravis, and multiple sclerosis, afflict women anywhere from two to 10 times more often than they do men.

Yes, our sex hormones, our x chromosomes, and a history of pregnancy all play a role in the development of autoimmune disease, but there are other important pieces to the autoimmune puzzle in women as well. One of those pieces is what I call the autoimmune mindset. The autoimmune mindset is formed in childhood and impacts your health in adulthood.

I am one of the 50 million Americans who has received an autoimmune diagnosis. I know what it's like to be trapped inside a sick body, a body in pain that is constantly exhausted. I know what happens when it seems your body has betrayed you. You can become depressed, you might reach for convenience foods that you think will provide comfort. If it hurts to move, you will stop moving. Then you might start gaining weight, becoming even more discouraged and even ashamed that you can't get a handle on your life. You might start going online to find a quick-fix diet solution. You may be too overwhelmed with fatigue to follow an eating plan that would help you, opting instead for easy-to-mix liquid diets.

Then there's the frustration that arises when you are eating and doing "everything right" and yet you still don't feel good. You might believe that your body has betrayed you and resent the hell out of it. You begin to think of your body as your adversary and of food as the enemy since you feel so terrible after every meal. You say words like, "I am struggling with my _____." Fill in the blank. It could be your weight, your energy level, your libido, your sleep, your skin, your mood, your menstrual cycle, your digestion, or your fertility if you are trying to conceive. You keep "fighting" against pain, brain fog, puffiness, and food cravings. This is the trap I found myself in twenty-five years ago. I found a way out and have written this book as a roadmap for you to find your way out too.

The road back from autoimmunity is not straight or without bumps and potholes. I am going to teach you a quick method for finding the missing pieces to your health puzzle. I am not going to fix you. I am going to provide the information you need to reverse your own autoimmunity.

There is no quick fix to ending autoimmune disease. If you have been exhausted, feeling sick for many years, and are even on multiple medications, I am telling you right now that you need to be patient. You can start feeling better quickly, but ending your autoimmunity can take a while. It requires patience and perseverance. I often observe women having far more patience and perseverance with people other than themselves. That is something we are going to work on together. You are worth persevering for, you deserve loving self-care, and the little child inside of you desperately wants you to be patient with her.

Please also keep in mind that if you already have an autoimmune disease, potentially with organ damage, it might have taken 10, 20, or even 30 years to develop. This is for certain; it did not happen "all of a sudden" or "overnight" the way most of us believe when we are diagnosed. That being said, it won't take decades for you to start feeling better, because I am giving you a quick-start program that will get you going on the right track as you learn to solve your own autoimmune puzzle. I am teaching you the method I have successfully used to end autoimmunity for hundreds of my patients. It is the method I created for myself.

What You Can Expect

As you learn and implement the method I have laid out for you, your symptoms of fatigue, pain, digestive problems, insomnia, anger, depression, anxiety, and inflammation will start to reduce within 7–10 days. You will start to see a change in your weight as you start to lose puffiness and swelling over the next 10–21 days. By the end of the month, your brain fog will have lifted, and any skin rashes you have will have reduced, if not disappeared. To make the math easier, expect a 50% reduction of symptoms over the next few weeks, provided you take the steps I describe. You will get out of this what you put into it.

Some of the tools I am teaching you will take time for you to practice as you learn to create new habits. You must schedule this time for yourself. I find that women with autoimmunity struggle with self-care, focusing instead on caring for others. This is a strategy you learned long ago that has kept you from learning to love yourself. When you compulsively care for everyone else and ignore your own body's feedback, this is not rooted in compassion. It's you helping others so you will feel worthy of even being alive.

I am saying very clearly to you, "I give you permission to take care of you. You are worth it and no one around you wants you to be sick." I wish someone had said those words to me in the years before I got so sick. When I tell you that caring for others and ignoring yourself is not love or compassion, that is fierce love from me as I speak my truth to you. You are a girl worth saving. Please listen. I once delivered this message to a dear friend of mine who was so busy caring for her mother, she was ignoring her own self-care. I asked her if she wanted her daughter to be in the same overscheduled, hamster-wheel hell she was in. She stopped, got tears in her eyes as the realization slowly sunk in that she was setting herself up to get very sick. The next caregiver in line was her only daughter. "Message received" was her quiet response.

The Method

You are going to learn how to **BRIDGE** the gap from where you are today to where you want to be. This means you will learn about your **B**rain, your **R**elay System (nervous system and hormone system), your **I**deas about yourself, your life experiences and the people you share your life with. You will learn the role **D**iet plays in your gut health. You will discover how the health of your **G**ut impacts your genetic expression and immune system. Finally, you will understand why your ability to **E**xcrete what you no longer need is so important (think about how essential it is to take out the trash). This **BRIDGE** is the foundation on which we will build and solve your autoimmune puzzle.

This is not the Standard American Medicine (SAM) model of healthcare you are used to that focuses on matching symptoms to drugs. Uncle SAM's healthcare model is great for acute emergencies. If you are having a heart attack, need to have a broken bone set, or urgently need your appendix out, please call Uncle SAM. But the Uncle SAM model is sorely lacking when it comes to preventing disease or ending autoimmune disease, which is what we are up to in this book.

The Freedom Framework
(the frame of your puzzle)

I am helping you **BRIDGE** the gap between disease and wellness. There are four pillars that hold your **BRIDGE** up. These are the four sides of your puzzle and the four steps of the method I am going to take you through that will help you reverse your autoimmunity. I call this four-step process the Freedom Framework. It is designed to take you from fatigue, pain, and inflammation to vitality and wellness. The four pillars of the Freedom Framework, *see figure 1*, can be applied to any autoimmune disease to get you from feeling awful to feeling like a human again.

The steps are:
1. un-**C**over root cause(s).
2. **C**onfront the data collected through laboratory testing and your own story.
3. **C**onnect your beliefs and behaviors with your current reality.
4. **C**reate the life you want to be living with full intention.

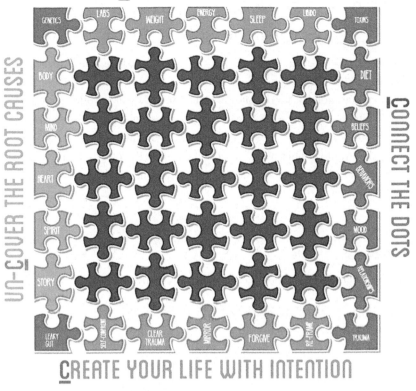

▲ Figure 1

The Freedom Framework with the four corner (root cause) pieces of the autoimmune puzzle

The BIG Pieces of the Puzzle (the corner pieces that anchor the whole thing together)

There are four corner pieces, *see figure 2*, to the puzzle of autoimmune disease we will be exploring together. These four corner pieces are scientifically validated common causes of autoimmune disease. I will introduce you to some of the studies as we explore each one. These will be the anchor pieces to your puzzle. They are: 1) your genetics, 2) environmental toxins, 3) leaky gut, and 4) trauma. This last piece of the puzzle is the one I call the missing piece. It's also the piece that I find my female patients are the most resistant to exploring.

▼ **Figure 2**

The 4 corner pieces, or root causes, of autoimmune disease

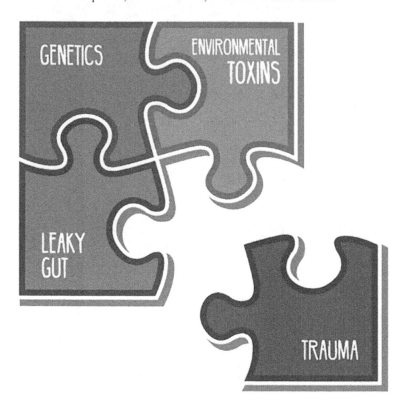

The Challenge

I will walk you through the Freedom Framework method using my own story and the stories of patients of mine who have also had their autoimmunity reversed. I have changed their names and some of the details of their stories to protect their privacy. You will see that each of these people has their own unique root causes that contributed to their autoimmunity, whether urticaria, mixed connective tissue disease, MS, eczema, or any number of other diseases. I will take you through a step-by-step method for finding the pieces that solved each of their health puzzles. All of them had previously been to doctor after doctor with no success in ending their diseases. This might be your story too. If you are puzzled about how to gain freedom from a body attacking itself, read on.

What This Book Is Not, and My Promise to You

This book is not just about food, supplements, and lab testing. These are certainly all part of your program, but in addition, you will learn what no other program is teaching:

- How to love yourself (flaws and all).
- How to set boundaries with the toxic people and experiences in your life.
- How to make friends with your body.
- How to reclaim your power and heal your inner self-saboteur if you have a history of childhood trauma.
- How to reframe self-limiting beliefs that keep you stuck in a victim story.

Ayurvedic medicine, the 5,000-year-old sister science of yoga, tells us that autoimmune disease is anger turned against oneself. Girls are often positively reinforced for being "good," "helpful," and "quiet." Women are considered aggressive, abrasive, and unfeminine when they express their feelings and speak their truth. If you have an autoimmune disease, you have a body attacking itself—no, killing itself. I am going to teach you to find the anger you have turned on yourself. You will see where you are blocking yourself from showing up as the brightest and shiniest version of yourself that you can be. And I am going to say right now, "How dare you deprive me of your light? Why do you think it's okay for others to do the work required to show up and you get to stay at home and go dark?"

That's me again with some fierce love for you! It's true. When you are not fully lit up, you are not contributing to the light required for us to succeed as a human species. All members of the team are required right now more than ever. It's time to play full out!

I've Got Your Back

As women, we are all different from one another. We have our own unique gene pool, our own life experiences, and our own definitions of what it means to be a woman in our contemporary world. This book outlines a method for understanding and solving your own unique puzzle and putting the pieces together in a way that matches *your* life. There is no "one-size-fits-all" pair of jeans or pair of genes. When you are finished with this program, you will know yourself better than anyone else knows you. You will know how to set boundaries with the toxins in your life (people and thoughts included). You will be powerful in mind, body, heart, and spirit. Will all of this happen by the end of this book? Perhaps, but not likely. However, you will be on your way.

Remember there is "we" in wellness and "I" in illness. I just want to say right now that I am proud of you. I am inspired by your courage and I know you are up to this challenge. You are never given any problem you are incapable of solving, though sometimes you will require some help from others. This is your next level of growth, and I am honored to walk with you on this journey. I have walked this path. Everything I teach here I do. I have not "cured" my autoimmune disease. I have "reversed" it. I have "ended" it. Why this distinction? Because if I went back to the diet, beliefs, behavior patterns and ways of dealing with stress and anger that I had when I was first diagnosed, I would once again activate the genes that put me at risk for RA in the first place.

But I am jumping ahead. Let me start at the beginning with my own story.

SECTION I:
The Puzzle

"Somebody once told me the definition of hell: On your last day on earth, the person you became will meet the person you could have become."

~ANONYMOUS

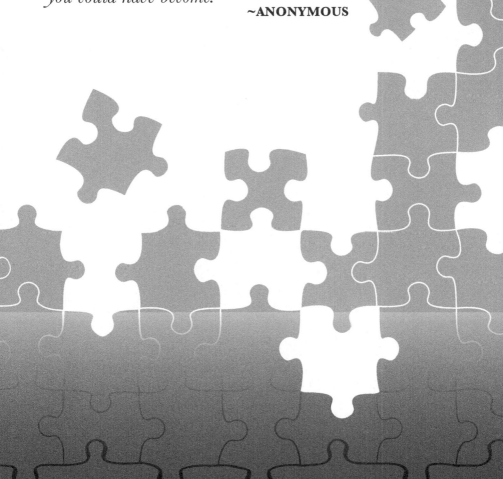

CHAPTER 1

My Personal Autoimmune Puzzle

"Although the world is full of suffering, it is also full of the overcoming of it."

~HELEN KELLER

An Incurable Wake-Up Call

When I was in my early 30s, I was diagnosed with rheumatoid arthritis (RA). RA is an autoimmune disease that is considered incurable. One day I was running marathons, working part time as a registered nurse in my local hospital, raising my four beautiful children, and preparing to take a family vacation to Florida. The next day I was aching with pain, could hardly move, and some of my joints were swollen and red. I went to see my doctor. After blood tests and x-rays, I was informed I had rheumatoid arthritis (RA). How, I wondered, did "all of a sudden" I develop RA when I exercised, ate home-cooked meals, and was healthy when compared to lots of people in my community? I will address this commonly asked question later in this book. To me, this was a puzzle that needed to be solved.

My doctor offered me a cancer-fighting drug and some strong anti-inflammatory drugs as "treatment." Since my grandfather had also had RA, my doctor told me it was likely genetic and shrugged her shoulders saying there was not much else to be discussed. I asked her if my diet had any impact on my genetics and inflammation. Was there something I could do besides take the drugs? She responded with a firm and very dismissive "no."

I went home and threw myself into research articles about RA on my computer. I was determined to solve this puzzle quickly. My first and foremost concern was my family. I was the primary caregiver in my household and my husband was the primary bread winner. How would my children fare if I was in constant pain? I was beset with anxiety on their behalf. My illness could change their lives, and it was not their fault.

I could feel my stomach tighten and my joint pain increase as my anxiety over the "what ifs" began to churn. What if I can't be present for my kids when they get home from school? How will they feel if I can't really listen to them recount the highs and lows of the day? What if I am not there with a healthy snack and warm smile to greet them after they have spent the day in the "social jungle" called elementary school? What if I can no longer help with homework or go on our weekly adventures together? What if we can't go hiking, bike riding, skiing together as a family any longer? My anxiety was doing nothing to ease my joint pain. I turned to a familiar refuge. I baked my favorite "comfort" food, chocolate chip cookies, to sustain me during what was turning out to be hours of reading research articles.

I had to stop my daily jogging because of my painful joints. I noticed my mood becoming jagged as irritability floated to the surface due to my lack of exercise. Running had been my one and only free time away from the responsibilities of child rearing. Deprived of my morning break, I was getting snappy and short tempered. I also felt impatient with the pain I was in. This was not my normal state of being. I was used to being called "the Energizer Bunny" and having endless energy. Now I was just exhausted. With my energy went my libido—both gone as the pain settled in. My self-image and self-worth were being affected—not by RA, but by the way I was responding to it.

I began gaining weight. I had never been thin as a child or as a teen. I had what I called a "normal" body type and had to exercise regularly to keep it that way. With my emotional distress, I started baking more of the foods I and my family loved. If my kids couldn't have a "fun and active mom" they could have a mom that kept them well-fed and happy with their favorite foods. Those foods were of course baked goods with plenty of sugar, chocolate, milk, and flour in them.

A Ray of Hope

Eventually, in my frantic research, I found an article about yoga as an "alternative treatment" for autoimmunity. I had not started the medications I had been prescribed because of the long list of potentially life-altering

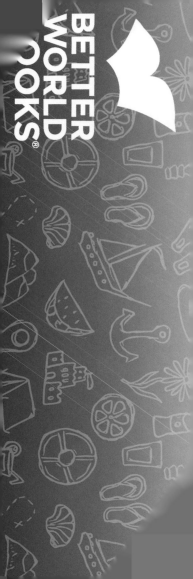

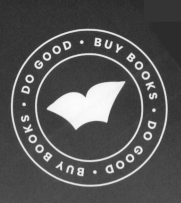

DO GOOD · BUY BOOKS ·
DO GOOD · BUY BOOKS ·

$35 million
raised for literacy

38 million
books donated

475 million
books reused or recycled

87 million
customers served

LEARN MORE

side effects they came with. As I munched an oatmeal chocolate-chip cookie and drank a glass of milk to wash it down with, I decided to go to my first yoga class.

During class the teacher asked us to leave our "egos at the door." He assured us they would be waiting there for us to pick them up again when we put our shoes on to leave. He also asked us to be present with only our bodies and our experiences, not to look around the room and compare ourselves to others who might be more flexible. Then he gave me the first puzzle piece to solving this new health crisis I was in. He mentioned the word Ayurveda.

Ayurveda, he said, was the sister science of yoga. It came from India and was a way of individualizing our daily routine. We all have different body types, and we all require different diets, sleep schedules, exercise programs, and learning methods. For me, this was revolutionary. I was a nurse, completely steeped in Western medicine. I had never considered anything beyond the food pyramid and the American Heart Association or the American Diabetic Association guidelines for food plans.

I went home and straight away got on the computer. To illustrate how long ago this was, I connected to the Internet via a dial-up modem. I used the search engine of the time called "Ask Jeeves" to ask about Ayurveda. I was filled with excitement, elation, and hope as I spent the next two hours reading about this 5,000-year-old science of living according to your unique constitutional type. I learned that these body types are called doshas. There are 3 constitutional types and they are known as vata, pitta, and kapha. I began studying up on my particular body type.

I soon discovered *why* I had RA. This had not been a question I had explored beyond the "Why me?" "Why now?" victimization level. It struck me that the why was the most important factor in getting to an actual cure rather than just "managing symptoms." I discovered that my inflammation was being aggravated by so many of my daily habits. Not only my daily routine, but the way I thought and the way I held onto frustration and anger.

Autoimmunity, from an Ayurvedic perspective, is undigested anger. I was not friends with the woman I saw in the mirror each day. Internally I was a war zone. I had an adversarial relationship with my body. I had spent most of my adult life trying to "beat it into shape" by literally pounding away over miles and miles of asphalt with my running shoes. I had starved it, hated it, berated it. I had even allowed others to cut out parts that I saw as responsible for causing me pain, such as my tonsils, varicose veins, and gall bladder.

This idea of inflammation and pain stemming from my food choices and my thoughts was new. This was revolutionary. This was mind blowing. Ayurveda was a whole new paradigm for me. I had to sit with it and process it. I took a meditation class and began meditating daily.

Death by Suicide

One day, as I was meditating, the word "autoimmune" entered my mind. As I sat, I began to think of it from different perspectives. The word auto-immune, I realized, meant I was attacking myself. I began self-inquiry along this line. Why was I attacking me? Why was I killing myself? My immune system was attacking me as if I were a virus or bacteria. Why was I not friends with myself? Asking the question "why" was the second piece of the puzzle that got me closer to understanding my health dilemma.

That day during meditation and self-inquiry, I followed the why question as if I was retracing my steps back through a labyrinth I had gotten lost in. I visualized a golden thread going back to my childhood and tried to find where it started. When did I decide to attack myself? When did I start viewing myself as a virus or bacteria that needed to be done away with?

Another Piece of the Puzzle Revealed

That thought thread led me back to being ten years old. I was a Navy brat and that meant I moved a lot. In fact, by the time I was fourteen, I had moved twenty-one times. I was extremely introverted and painfully shy. Then, when I was in fourth grade, I started getting called into one of the school administrator's offices.

I thought I was in trouble when my name was first called out over the intercom in my class to go to the office. I was embarrassed and scared. What had I done? I had never been called into a school office and was known in my other schools and at home as being a "good and well-behaved girl." It happened repeatedly. The first few times I was called to this administrator's office, he just talked to me about behaving in class. I stammered that I was behaving and he let me return to class. Nonetheless, whenever the intercom rang in the classroom, I felt my heart race and my breathing grow shallow and fast. My hands got clammy as I clutched the number 2 pencil, and the green lines on the tan sheet of paper began to blur.

The Monster in the Shadow

As you may have guessed, these visits to the office turned into something other than talk. He began sexually abusing me and telling me that if I wasn't good, I would be back "for more." I tried to tell the playground teachers. I went to my class teacher as well. Nobody listened. When I approached my mother, who also failed to comprehend the gravity of the situation, she told me to keep "my nose down" and do good work. My father likewise told me to "use protective camouflage and blend in" and "when in Rome learn to get along with the Romans." He said I needed to learn to get along with people that were different than me; he approached it like it was a racial issue. I was one of two Caucasian girls in my school.

I began experiencing headaches and stomach pain every morning when I woke up. I didn't want to go to school anymore. This was unusual because in spite of my shyness, I was an insatiable reader and learner and absolutely loved school. I had always been a good student with no prior attempts of ditching school. I started gaining weight and using sugar as comfort food. My mom was a great baker and we usually had some form of homemade treat cooling on the countertop in the kitchen after school. These gluten and sugar-filled treats became my solace.

Finding the Light

I started spending a lot of time by myself on our balcony under the coconut tree that grew in the front of our apartment building. I sat out there to get away from everyone, so I could just stare at the clouds and pray. When I was alone, I could feel the presence of angels. I knew I was loved and being watched over, in spite of my experiences at school. When I was on the balcony, I began talking to these warm, glowing beings of light. I told them I would rather be with them. I wanted to "come home." I was finding planet earth too dangerous and difficult to navigate. I asked for a ticket out.

I began seeing myself "dying young." I started telling my parents I would never be a grandmother. I knew I would not live to an old age. I had it from the mouth of angels that I could leave in a few more years. I began to see the end of my life as freedom from the trap I was in. I was not friends with the girl I saw in the mirror each morning. After all, she was clearly "bad" or she wouldn't be in so much trouble all the time. She was also obviously "invisible and not important" or people would listen to her plea for protection. These distorted beliefs, made up due to trauma I could not understand, are another piece of the puzzle of my autoimmunity.

Heeding the Call

Flash forward to my 30s during my meditation, sitting on my cushion. My eyes flew open as the realization hit me squarely between the eyes. At ten years old, I had decided that death was the only way out of a terrible situation. This conclusion had been recorded in my cells and then impacted my genetic expression. It had activated my family history of RA.

As I began to implement a new lifestyle, I soon discovered there were several other pieces to this puzzle. I had been exposed to second-hand cigarette smoke in my childhood. I was treated for frequent urinary tract infections with antibiotics early in my life. I was also prescribed antibiotics multiple times in my adolescent years to treat cases of strep throat. I was addicted to sugar and ate it disguised as "healthy" homemade treats, which also contained gluten and dairy, both of which (I later discovered through functional medicine testing) I am quite intolerant to. I used over-the-counter Ibuprofen frequently to get me through my marathon training and running schedule.

Then there was the emotional and psychological side. I was a perfectionist and drove myself hard throughout my early teen and adult years. I was also a harsh judge of myself and others and did not forgive readily. I held onto the hurts of the past, erroneously thinking that keeping them close would protect me from being hurt again.

But the missing piece to this puzzle, the one that reversed my autoimmune disease for good, was the realization that I believed I was not worth protecting. I was not safe, and I was not loveable unless I was perfect. I had what I now call an "autoimmune mindset." This is a state of such overwhelm, such busyness, such striving for improvement, that the body has to scream to get your attention.

I had early warnings, soft whispers from my body. I had acne in my teens that I took Accutane for. I got extremely nauseated when I went on the oral contraceptive pill. I struggled with my weight. I had terrible brain fog. My knees began to ache. My moods went crazy before I started my periods. I craved sugar every afternoon. I woke up tired every morning and fought to get out of bed. Each and every one of these issues are part of the same root cause, and all of them were warning signs from my body that things were imbalanced and getting worse.

Like many of my patients, I took a medication to solve the symptom. This did not solve the root issue, it just made my body have to turn up the volume. When did I finally pay attention? When my pain was so great I couldn't move. When my joints were angry and red and inflamed. When I was diagnosed with RA. My puzzle was starting to take shape, and I was finally ready to look at the pieces and the whole picture.

Within one year of implementing the method I am laying out for you here, my RA was reversed. It has now been over twenty years since I have had any sign of my autoimmune disease. This is not the normal trajectory of RA in the Western medicine paradigm. In fact, as my doctor had told me, it's considered incurable.

Healing the Whole Person

I knew the reversal of my disease was so dramatic because I had been willing to explore my mental health, emotional health, physical health, and spiritual health. I had heeded the call, examined my story, and found the meanings that had been made up by an upset 10-year old. I saw the beliefs I had made up as a child and discovered the self-limiting behaviors I had adopted as a result. These were literally killing me. I transformed my life and habits completely in all 5 of these areas (mind, emotions, body, spirit, and story). I discovered and applied for myself the Freedom Framework— the very same method for finding and fixing the root sources of dis-ease that I am presenting to you in this book.

Not long after making my Ayurveda-inspired lifestyle changes, I discovered functional medicine. I realized this was a model that took some of the precepts of Ayurveda and translated them into Western language for the modern person. The synthesis of my 30+ years of education and clinical expertise is now integrated into this book, which we will explore together, piece by piece.

In my work with my patients, I have discovered that no two puzzles are the same. Each person has their own genetic makeup, their own toxic exposure, their own lives and stories. I have also discovered just how much courage it takes to have the willingness to confront the long-held beliefs you created in childhood that have now become your strategies in life. These beliefs have informed behaviors that are now your habits.

The energy that motivates your thoughts and your deeds was framed in your childhood. Imagine, all of us running around in adult bodies with childish beliefs. It's why we get into so much conflict in our relationships, in the workplace, and in the world. The great news is that if you are reading this book, you now have an adult brain. You can reflect on those early meanings you made up so long ago and actually change them if they are not serving you. Possessing the willingness and courage to self-confront and look at all of the pieces to your puzzle is the only requirement to gain freedom from suffering. This is the only way out of autoimmunity.

No One-Size-Fits-All Cure for Anything

We are not "standardized" people and so there can never be standardized interventions for what we want to think of as standard problems. There is no such thing. This is the lie of "evidence-based medicine." Our scientific research is done on random samplings of small groups of the population and then we attempt to extrapolate data that we can apply to everyone. That is why the list of side effects for every medication ever invented is so long. We react to our food, medications, sleep, exercise, thoughts, experiences, climate, age, and toxins very differently. There is no diet that will solve autoimmunity for every person. There is no therapist who will be right for everyone. Everything must be individualized to fit you as the unique person you are.

Health *and* dis-ease are both byproducts of your genetics plus your physical, mental, and emotional digestive health. Vitality is a result of your exposure to toxins of all kinds, and your ability to detoxify or rid yourself of the toxins you have been exposed to. It is a result of your ability to assimilate the nutrients from your food, thoughts, and emotions and to eliminate what you do not need. This process leads to vitality, or what I think of as life force.

The remainder of this book will be about finding the pieces to your puzzle. It is a scientifically proven method that will help you gain freedom from your suffering. We will take a journey through the 4 pillars of the Freedom

Framework. Each step along your **BRIDGE** is meant to empower you to heal yourself.

I am providing you with a set of instructions for how to put your puzzle together so you don't have to wander around desperately trying to find answers to why you are still trapped by your weight, your hormones, autoimmune disease, your lack of energy and vitality, low libido, mood swings, digestive issues, heart problems, blood sugar imbalances, thyroid disorders, infertility, menstrual problems, and any other pain you are experiencing. Autoimmunity takes many shapes; hence, why there are so many kinds of puzzles.

Let's start with the big picture on the front of the box before we dump all the puzzle pieces out on the table.

CHAPTER 2

The Big Picture

"It's always the small pieces that make the big picture."

~UNKNOWN

Why Autoimmunity is a Puzzle

The word "autoimmune" means that your immune system has begun to attack you. Autoimmunity means your immune system has lost the ability to differentiate between you and the foreign invaders it is designed to protect you from, such as bacteria, fungi, parasites, and viruses. An autoimmune disease develops when your immune system, which defends your body against disease, decides your healthy cells are foreign. As your hyper-vigilant immune system attacks healthy cells and body tissue, you can end up with damaged organs and body systems and ultimately cancer, even death.

The American Autoimmune Related Disease Association (AARDA) reports there are 50 million Americans who have one or more autoimmune diseases, and that number is rising. Autoimmune illnesses are the second most common cause of chronic illness in the United States after heart disease. Researchers have identified over 145 different autoimmune diseases and that number is also rising. I am not alone in considering this one of the most alarming health crises of our time.

Autoimmune diseases will often fluctuate between remission, with little or no symptoms, and flares that include worsening of symptoms. The SAM model focuses on relieving symptoms by using toxic prescription drugs and over-the-counter medications. The commonly used immunosuppressant treatments and non-steroidal anti-inflammatory drugs (NSAIDs) used as pain relievers lead to devastating long-term side effects while making the pharmaceutical industry millions, if not billions of dollars a year.

Because many autoimmune diseases have similar symptoms, people can go for years undiagnosed. In the current SAM model of matching drugs to symptoms, the vague and often overlapping symptoms have made diagnosis difficult and medical delivery of care convoluted in the extreme. When you develop one autoimmune disease, you are 75% likely to develop another, and another. Why? Because we are not addressing the root causes of autoimmunity. We are chasing symptoms, and people are getting sicker and sicker and dying because of a healthcare paradigm that is not working.

One Bucket with Many Disease Names

More and more diseases are being classified as autoimmune as our understanding of the immune system and its interplay with genetics broadens. Often my patients will come to my office with the misinformed idea that their autoimmune disease originates in the body tissue the immune system is attacking. For example, rheumatoid arthritis originates in the joints, or Hashimoto's thyroiditis originates in the thyroid. This is not correct, and we will get into more detail on this in Chapter 5 when we explore leaky gut.

Autoimmune disease is a disease of an immune system that has become hyper-vigilant. Because 70% of the immune system is contained in the gut, having a healthy digestive system is essential. This is one of the root causes we will discuss in Chapter 5.

First let's talk about the growing number of autoimmune diseases. There are over 145 identified autoimmune diseases and the list is growing all the time as more and more research places known diseases in the autoimmune bucket (*see Figure 3*). Type 2 diabetes mellitus, now considered an autoimmune disease, is a great example of this reclassification.

Table 1 consists of some common autoimmune diseases I see in my practice. It is by no means exhaustive.

We now know cardiovascular diseases and cancers have an autoimmune component too. Aren't these diseases genetic? Yes, as are over one-third of autoimmune diseases. This places more and more emphasis on keeping your gut healthy and the microbes that are impacting how your genetics are expressed diverse. More on this in Chapters 5 and 7.

All autoimmune diseases can go into the same bucket since they are all diseases of a hyper-vigilant immune system, not the target organs.

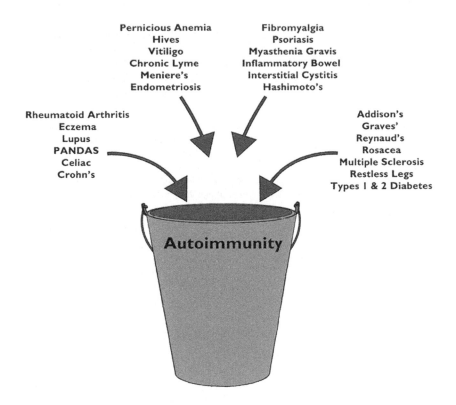

What Are Typical Symptoms of Autoimmune Disease?

At this point you can see that the symptoms of autoimmune disease are as varied as the target organ the immune system has begun to attack. However, remember that autoimmune disease is a result of several root causes that have usually been actively out of balance for a long time before diagnosis. Before full blown disease, there are usually warning signs of worsening imbalance. One of the most common signs your body gives you that something is wrong is fatigue. We women don't usually tolerate fatigue and our "no pain no gain" work ethos can drive us to reach for a caffeinated

▼ Table 1: Autoimmune diseases

AUTOIMMUNE DISEASE	SYMPTOMS/COMMENTS
Rheumatoid arthritis	Causes inflammation of the joints and surrounding tissues.
Eczema	Patches of dry, itchy skin that worsen and erupt into rash (and sometimes become infected) as they are scratched.
Systemic lupus erythematosus	Can affect the skin, joints, kidneys, brain, and other organs. Symptoms depend on the organ(s) affected.
PANDAS *(pediatric autoimmune neuropsychiatric disorders associated with streptococcus)*	I am seeing more and more children in my practice who have been diagnosed with PANDAS. It is a term used to describe children who get a "sudden onset" of symptoms, such as compulsive behavior, motor tics, and anxiety following an infection.
Celiac sprue disease	A reaction to gluten that causes damage to the lining of the small intestine and can target multiple organs and tissues in the body.
Crohn's disease	An inflammatory bowel disease characterized by persistent inflammation of the lining of the gastrointestinal tract.
Pernicious anemia	A decrease in red blood cells caused by inability to absorb vitamin B-12.
Autoimmune urticaria	Chronic hives.
Vitiligo	White patches on the skin caused by loss of pigment.
Chronic Lyme disease	An inflammatory disease caused by Borrelia burgdorferi bacteria and believed to be autoimmune related.
Meniere's disease	A disorder of the inner ear.
Scleroderma	A connective tissue disease that causes changes in skin, blood vessels, muscles, and internal organs.
Endometriosis	Occurs when the kind of tissue that normally lines a woman's uterus grows on the ovaries, behind the uterus, or on the bowels or bladder. This can cause pain, infertility, and very heavy periods.
Fibromyalgia	A chronic disorder characterized by widespread pain, tenderness, and fatigue.

AUTOIMMUNE DISEASE	SYMPTOMS/COMMENTS
Psoriasis	A skin condition that causes redness and irritation as well as thick, flaky, silver-white patches.
Psoriatic arthritis	In addition to the skin disorder, people with psoriatic arthritis also have pain, stiffness, and swelling of the joints.
Myasthenia gravis	Muscle weakness.
Inflammatory bowel diseases	A group of inflammatory diseases of the colon and small intestine.
Interstitial cystitis	Chronic bladder pain.
Hashimoto's disease	Inflammation of the thyroid gland.
Addison's disease	Adrenal hormone insufficiency.
Mixed connective tissue disease	Called the overlap disease because it is characterized by signs and symptoms of a combination of disorders—primarily lupus, scleroderma, and polymyositis.
Graves' disease	Characterized by an overactive thyroid gland.
Reynaud's disease	Cold fingertips.
Reactive arthritis	Inflammation of the joints, urethra, and eyes; may cause sores on the skin and mucus membranes.
Rosacea	Rash on the face characterized by redness, bumpy texture of skin, acne, and swelling.
Sjögren's syndrome	Destroys the glands that produce tears and saliva causing dry eyes and mouth; may affect kidneys and lungs.
Multiple sclerosis	Disease of the nervous system that affects the brain and the spinal cord.
Restless leg syndrome	When the legs become uncomfortable in any position and cannot be kept still. It can be accompanied by a sensation of creeping, crawling, tingling, or burning.
Type 1 diabetes	Destruction of insulin-producing cells in the pancreas.
Type 2 diabetes	Type 2 diabetes is in the process of being redefined as an autoimmune disease rather than just a metabolic disorder.

beverage, pill, or a sugar-packed food source rather than have our forward motion impeded. We have been telling ourselves that we have to bring home the bacon, fry it up in a pan, and look hot at the same time. This need to look like Super Woman is destroying the male/female balance on the planet, and it is literally killing each of us as we develop autoimmunity and cancer in numbers never before known in our history.

This compulsive self-drive is dangerous behavior. If you are consistently tired, and you have been getting 8 hours of sleep a night, it's time to ask your body what it needs. After you ask, it's important to listen. These are basic rules of functional, healthy communication. Relationships between people are not healthy when one person gets tuned out, ignored, talked over, and avoided.

John Gottman, one of the leading experts on marriage and relationships, tells us that relationships that are not based on trust, healthy communication, and active listening will not last. This goes for your relationship with your body too. The relationship won't last if you are not listening. Your body will walk out on you if you deem everything else in your life as more important. You cannot have an affair with your coffee cup, your computer, your schedule, your to-do list, etc. and expect your body to stay quiet. Just like any marriage, it takes mindful attention and a lot of work to keep it healthy. This is the same with the marriage between your mind, your heart, your body, and your spirit. Is it filing for divorce or do you still get along?

Some early warning signs of autoimmune disease are:
- Fatigue
- Brain fog (difficulty focusing, concentrating, and remembering)
- Hair loss
- Digestive issues such as constipation, abdominal cramping, diarrhea, bloating, gas
- Numbness or tingling in the hands, feet, or face
- Dry eyes, mouth, or skin
- Muscle weakness
- Joint pain
- Rashes, hives, itchy skin or ears
- Infertility and miscarriages
- Unexplained weight gain or loss
- Fever
- Menstrual cycle changes
- General malaise (feeling ill)

Autoimmune diseases affect many parts of the body. Remember, auto-immune diseases develop when your immune system attacks healthy cells. Your immune system is designed to defend you against diseases caused by bacteria, fungi, parasites, and viruses. The healthy cells and organ systems it is attacking determine how your autoimmune disease will be diagnosed and classified. Depending on the disease, your immune system can attack one or many different types of body tissue, putting you at risk for organ damage.

The most common tissues and organ systems affected are the:
- Skin
- Joints
- Endocrine or hormone system
- Red blood cells and blood vessels
- Connective tissue
- Muscles

Who Gets Autoimmune Disease?

Anyone, from children to adults of all ethnicities, can get autoimmune disease. Women are at higher risk than men for developing autoimmunity; in fact, 80% of all autoimmune illnesses are diagnosed in women. Auto-immune disease is one of the top 10 leading causes of death in girls and women in all age groups up to 64 years of age.

In my clinical practice, I diagnose autoimmune diseases daily in people who had no idea that they had a health issue that has a name, let alone is an autoimmune disease. Some great examples of this are Raynaud's disease, eczema, rosacea, and restless leg syndrome. Often my patients with the tell-tale blue fingers of Raynaud's disease will respond to my inquiry about their finger color with, "Oh this just happens when I get too cold." Or when I comment on a new patient's peeling, red, rashy hands I hear, "Oh, that just happens sometimes; it's not there all of the time. I just use a little steroid cream and it disappears." The rest of that sentence is, "and it comes back when I stop using the steroid cream."

Taking a steroid to keep inflammation under control is not getting to the root of the problem. In fact, it's making it worse by aggravating the lining of the gut even more. Usually my patients with these issues that are their "normal" don't even realize they are autoimmune. They have never heard of leaky gut and have certainly never tried to get to the root causes of their leaky gut. Their doctors have given them things to manage the surface symptoms. Meanwhile, the actual root problems are getting worse and worse.

The Link Between Stress and Your Immune System

I will be talking a lot about the impact of distressing life events from your childhood; how these have impacted your genetic expression and how the stress from these events affects your gut health and subsequently your immune system. An impaired digestive tract leaves you open to environmental triggers such as bacteria, viruses, fungi, parasites, molds, chemicals, and estrogen-mimicking pollutants. It's all connected, and each piece of the puzzle is important. Stress is a misunderstood factor in the development of autoimmunity, so I am going to take some time here to clarify its role.

The 4F Stress Response System

Over 80% of people diagnosed with autoimmune disease report a subjective impression of emotional stress before the onset of their symptoms. I would say 100% of my patients report feeling overwhelmed in some way when they come to see me with fatigue, weight issues, gut problems, pain, hormone imbalances, memory loss, and inflammation. Their perception of their stress is high when they are imbalanced.

I am going to introduce you to a lot of "f words" in this section. Having fun with the letter "f" will help you to remember just how stress impacts your health. Your body's stress response system, known as the *4F stress response system* or sympathetic nervous system, responds to your *perceptions* of stress. I am going to refer to the *4F stress response system* or sympathetic nervous system from now on as the *4F stress response system*. The 4F stress response system is activated when you perceive yourself to be in danger. This response interferes with your ability to feed, focus, forgive, and mate. (You get the picture about that last "f" word.)

In other words, you are unable to digest your food, thoughts, or emotions properly. Your mind narrows its perceptual lens when you feel stressed so that the only details you can take in are related to survival. When you are reacting from the 4F stress response system, you have activated your reptilian brain, which is unable to forgive, have fun, be friendly, have faith, flourish, or engage in functional relating with other human beings. In other words, when you are in a fury or a flurry of frazzled frustration, you will end up fatigued, fried, fat, frigid, frail, forlorn, fickle, and feel like a failure as you fling yourself into formulaic plans with fleeting, feeble rewards and fiddle fruitlessly with diets and pills, becoming fixated on the foolish fallacy that fast fixes with financial repercussions will free you from your brain fog and a body that feels like it's on the fritz. *Phew!*

The whole point of this book is to provide you with a framework that can help you find and fix the root causes that are blocking your flow, so that you can be free to fiercely flourish as the woman you are meant to be. You are a fascinating, fabulous female, who deserves to forge forward with fearless, fluid flexibility, saying farewell to fatalistic self-limiting beliefs forever. Okay, enough fun with "f words."

Stress is Not Bad for You

We often hear that stress is bad for you. You might have heard that stress is the cause of all illness. This is not true. It's your *perception* of your stress, your belief that the stress level you have is not manageable, that activates the 4F response system.

You actually need stress in your life. You need just *enough* stress to keep you challenged and motivated. It's when you perceive your challenges as overwhelming—too overwhelming to handle—that your immune system is impacted and you create what I call the autoimmune mindset. If you are anxious that you cannot meet the challenges you are presented with, your body will move into survival mode. The autoimmune mindset impacts your immune system. The perception of "too much stress" can flood your system with "too much cortisol" and create "too much reactivity" in your immune system. You wind up with leaky gut and all of the other issues that follow, as seen in *Figure 4*.

Have you ever had the experience that you might not even survive the level of stress you have in your life? I certainly have. This is when my breathing becomes shallow, I wake up in the night with my heart pounding, my belly feels like it has a giant knot in it, and I have an elephant on my chest. When you are perceiving your stress as insurmountable, your brain sends a message—using the messenger chemicals or hormones called neurotransmitters—that alerts the stress response system to get you to safety.

▼ **Figure 4**

Adrenal glands leaking cortisol lead to leaky gut which leads to autoimmunity and inflammatory problems of all kinds.

Adrenal System and Immune System

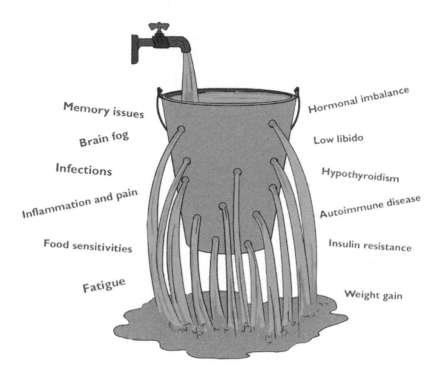

You are wired to be able to fight or run like crazy away from any threat to your survival. You will be like a zebra who has a lion on your tail who wants to eat you for lunch (*see figure 5*). Your heart rate will increase, your blood pressure will rise, your digestive system will shut down (not safe to stop and have a bowel movement if you have a hungry lion on your tail), and the hormones necessary for you to feel sexual desire will be reallocated to your survival system (also not safe to stop and reproduce if you are in danger of being eaten). Your muscles will then get the needed oxygenated blood for fleeing from the lion (or in this case your perceived lion), fighting it off, playing dead by freezing, or outright fainting. These messages and responses are the first two parts of the **BRIDGE**. I am talking about your **b**rain and your **r**elay system.

▼ Figure 5

Are you a zebra being chased by a lion and afraid you are going to be eaten for lunch?

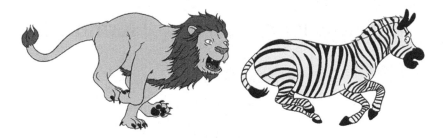

Your hormones relay the messages from the brain to tell the rest of the body what to do next. If you are sending stress signals from the brain, they will be relayed to the adrenal glands. The adrenal glands sit on top of your kidneys. The adrenal glands release a stress hormone called cortisol when they receive a danger signal from the brain.

Cortisol is a hormone. Almost every cell contains receptors for cortisol, so cortisol will behave according to the cell it's acting upon. When cortisol is balanced, it will help control blood-sugar levels, fluid balance, help you wake up in the morning, reduce inflammation, help with memory, and aid in fertility and blood pressure regulation. Cortisol, like stress, is not *bad*.

Too much cortisol can be damaging. When you are chronically releasing cortisol because you are chronically overwhelmed and chronically sending danger messages through your relay system, you will start seeing tissue and organ breakdown in your body, as well as weight gain and a decrease in your libido. This is one of the root causes of leaky gut. Cortisol breaks down the protective lining of your intestinal wall. Prolonged cortisol release can interfere with sleep or cause you to wake up fatigued in the morning even if you did get 8 hours of sleep. It can cause weight gain in the belly area, even when you are exercising and eating well. It affects your immune system, contributes to joint pain and inflammation, tanks your libido level, and can cause anxiety and depression—all of which are common symptoms in autoimmune disease as well. Adrenal fatigue is a primary cause of hormone imbalance in both men and women (*see figure 6*).

The Stress Response and How it Impacts Your Hormones

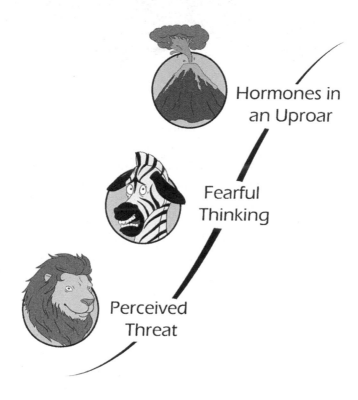

Hormones in an Uproar

Fearful Thinking

Perceived Threat

The 4F Life-Support System

You are wired to go into the 4F stress response system when there is danger or when you perceive danger, just as a zebra does when being chased by a lion. This allows you to respond instantly to a clear threat to your survival. Your body is then meant to go back into balance after you have gotten to safety, just like the zebra's does. When you are out of danger, you can then activate your 4F life-support system, which is necessary for proper digestion and assimilation of nutrients, fertility and reproduction, a healthy body mass index and weight, and the complete excretion of toxins from your mind and body. Unfortunately, in our fast-paced, productivity-oriented culture, we are not getting enough time to *rest and digest* or *feed and breed*, because we are hanging out in the *4F stress response system* so much of the time. I cannot count how many of my patients break down and cry or get outright angry with me when I suggest self-care activities designed to tone their 4F life-support system.

Important note: if you feel like crying or biting my head off when I tell you to add one more thing to your schedule, you have adrenal fatigue.

Here's what I know is true. If you feel stressed about scheduling some time every single day to take care of yourself, you have an autoimmune mindset and are either on your way to autoimmune disease or you already have one, if not more. And I am not talking about going to the gym as a method of self-care. If you are going to the gym and raising your heart rate, what is the message your body is getting? Is there a lion behind you causing you to run on that treadmill? Is the world going to end and that's why you are building your strength with weights? Your body cannot tell the difference between running for pleasure and running from danger. The same physiological changes occur, regardless of the motivation.

Exercise is necessary to keep your cardiovascular system healthy, your mood stable, your hormones balanced, to help you sleep soundly, and all of the other good and essential things it accomplishes. But here's the rub. If your adrenal glands are tired because you have been over-scheduled, over-stressed, over-care-giving, and over-achieving for a decade or more, then over-training is not going to get you feeling better. It's making you worse. It's causing your gut wall to break down. It's creating autoimmunity in your body.

Your body is attacking you to get your attention so you will stop CrossFit and listen to what it needs. Again, CrossFit is not bad. It's just not right for you if you are in a more advanced stage of adrenal fatigue usually present when you have an autoimmune disease. Am I telling you to become a slug, a couch potato, or a lazy person? No. This is not your ticket to stop exercising or to continue a potentially lethal sedentary lifestyle. It's me telling you to do what your body can manage right now. As you heal your adrenal and hormone system and your gut, you will be able to return to more strenuous exercise routines. Your exercise routine must match your body's needs. I will talk more about this in Section 3 as we start putting the puzzle pieces together.

Toning Your 4F Life-Support System Through Self-Care

The 4F life-support system helps you to be well-fed, fertile, friendly, and fearless. I am going to call it the 4F life-support system. We are microcosms of the macrocosm, and in order to support life, the entire interdependent web of life we live in as humans must be attended to. Without the proper assimilation of nutrients and elimination of toxins, you die. Without the ability to reproduce, we as a species dies. Without healthy communities, from the microcosmic cellular and microbiome ecosystems, to human societies, to planetary ecosystems, to the macrocosmic galaxies, we die. If you are chronically hanging out in the 4F stress response system day in and day out, you will die. Naturally, no one makes it out of this lifecycle without dying. However, by toning your 4F life-support system, you can enjoy your time on planet earth with more vitality and keep your mind and body healthier for longer.

When I talk about self-care and toning the 4F life-support system, I am talking about *really* connecting to your body, in a way that lets it know you are not in danger. Your mind knows you don't have a lion on your tail, but does your body? For every 5 minutes you are emotionally upset, it can take up to 8 hours for your body to recover and return to balance. Read that sentence again. When I learned that little mathematical formula, I was blown away. Boy was I in debt to my body! Really? Every 5-minute segment of hormonal craziness and mood swinging? YIKES! I didn't have enough 8-hour increments left in my lifetime to make that up. So I learned ways to speed up the process. Those are what I am going to teach you.

When I talk about self-care and toning your 4F life-support system, I am talking about letting your body know you are safe. I am not talking about getting a pedicure or a massage or going on vacation with girlfriends or sleeping in. These are all great activities. But they are not *toning* your 4F life-support system. They are dropping you into relaxation, but as soon as you are done with them, you are back into your prior autoimmune mindset.

The kind of self-care I am talking about is developing an intentional connection with your body. It's leaving behind the adversarial nature of your relationship with your schedule, your diet, your body, and your relationships and creating a collaborative alliance between your body, your heart, your mind, and your spirit. This requires being present with your body, not medicating it, numbing it, beating it, ignoring it, or talking badly to it or about it. It's bringing yourself into a state of acceptance, love, compassion, trust, and healthy communication with it.

This requires the development of self-awareness. That is what you will learn in this book. I not only didn't know how to do this when I was diagnosed with RA, I didn't even know I needed it. I was not self-aware enough to realize that my *perceptions* of stress, the way I dealt with my past hurts, and the behaviors that I had created as habits to deal with my emotions (like eating sugar and running long miles) were literally killing me.

Hanging Out in the Silence with You

After I had been practicing yoga and meditation for a few months, I came across a book that mentioned Vipassana meditation. Vipassana retreats, when done correctly, are no less than 10 days for beginners. Those 10 days are spent in nearly total silence that don't allow for eye contact with the other participants, let alone conversations. Not only that, but you are not permitted to have your cell phone, your journal, anything to read, outside food or drink, your yoga practice, your exercise program, or any other methods of self-soothing you might have. I can tell you that I had no idea just how disconnected I was from myself until I had to spend 10 days with just me, myself, and I…no interruptions! I found I didn't do anything mindfully. I didn't eat mindfully, shower mindfully, walk mindfully, parent mindfully, love my husband mindfully, think mindfully (sounds funny doesn't it?), or communicate with my body mindfully.

I am a hard nut who took a long time to crack. But by day three of my first Vipassana retreat, crack I did. At first I was angry. The stored anger I had from years of held-onto emotional pain bubbled up so I had to look at it. I discovered that if I didn't pay attention to the anger I was feeling, my back would ache to the point that I couldn't sit still. I went through layers of emotional upheaval during days three and four. In fact, on my solitary walks during the breaks we had from sitting, I wrote an entire book about Vipassana in my head. It was called, *Everything You Need to Know About Vipassana Meditation That No One Told You*. It was a scorcher, let me tell you.

Then on day five, I began to settle into the process. I was more willing and able to observe what came up, how it felt in my body, and then I figured out how to release it. Those of us that lasted through the entire 10 days found that we didn't want to talk when we were free to do so. We had each discovered the value of connection to the inner world and felt resistant to reconnecting to the outer world through idle chit chat.

I discovered just how out of touch with myself I had been for most of my life and realized this had played a large part in the development of my RA. I knew I had ignored the early warning signs my body had given me (like fatigue, acne, PMS, gall bladder disease, constipation, infections, joint pain, and an irregular menstrual cycle and lack of ovulation) and could have prevented the disease itself if I had been in the right relationship with my body and mind earlier. I also knew that everything happens in the timing that I am ready for it to happen. I now call this the misery-to-motivation ratio.

MISERY:MOTIVATION

The Misery-to-Motivation Ratio

People are willing to change their self-sabotaging behaviors to the degree that those behaviors are making them miserable. I have found this to be consistently true. I began noticing that my patients who were only mildly miserable were only willing to produce a mild effort to reverse their auto-immunity. The example I gave earlier about Raynaud's disease is perfect. It's easier to put some gloves on than it is to change your diet if your fingers are cold—unless you make the connection between your cold fingers and your gut and genetics. If you know those cold fingers are a harbinger of future disease, it can be more motivating. (But if you're not miserable yet, it probably won't be.)

My patients who come in whose sleep is tortured because of itchy skin, anxiety, or heart palpitations are desperate to do whatever it takes to sleep again. Those who cannot stand to even feel the fabric of their clothing against their skin because of hives are willing and ready to do whatever it takes to feel "normal" once again. Those who are in constant pain and can no longer engage in the activities they once enjoyed with the people they love are motivated to do whatever they need to do to feel alive again. Some are motivated by the desire to play with grandchildren. Others want to go back to work, to hike again, to dance again, even to walk again. When I was diagnosed with RA, my motivator was not only my lack of energy and joint pain, but I also wanted my children to be raised by a fully present and vibrant mother.

Find Your Why

My why has evolved over the last 20 years. It's what keeps me from reverting back to old destructive habits. I want to make sure I am not visited by the version of myself that I could have been and find that I have not met my potential. For me, not reaching my potential means I have wasted this lifetime. If I am not utterly grateful and appreciative for the life I have been granted, willing to take care of this amazing gift that is my body, and constantly challenging myself to utilize the gifts God has sent me here to share with my fellow beings, then I have not lived my purpose. That is my why for continuing to reframe and refine my beliefs, behaviors, and habits. It's to make sure I can shine a light for others who are floundering in the darkness of autoimmunity where I once was. This has taken me from an autoimmune mindset to a vitality mindset. I am no longer resistant to doing whatever it takes for me to expand and evolve and to help others do the same.

I encourage you to find your why. It's what will motivate you to make the life changes you will be challenged to make by this book. It's so much easier to reach for a chocolate-chip cookie than to develop self-awareness when you are overwhelmed. Believe me, I know. I am hoping that you will not have to get to rock bottom misery before you are motivated to make the changes you need to make in order to be the most brilliant and vital version of yourself you are meant to be.

It took me a long time and several hard lessons to learn how to love myself and to accept life as it shows up. I am going to teach you some tools for getting in touch with your body, for learning how to love yourself, and for toning your 4F life-support system. Let's start with a simple breathing exercise that will help you tone your 4F life-support system.

Tone Your Parasympathetic Nervous System

You now know the role stress plays in illness and disease. Remember also that for every 5 minutes you are in fight or flight, it takes your body 8 HOURS to recover. That may seem an overwhelming proportion, but there is yet hope to recover, because there are techniques to shorten that recovery time. Perhaps the simplest of these is conscious breathing. In Ayurveda and

Yoga, it's called pranayama. To really understand pranayama—why and how it works—is beyond the scope of our current discussion, but for now, you can think of it as conscious, yogic breathing. My favorite such exercise, because it is so simple yet effective, is 3-part yogic breathing.

3-Part Yogic Breathing

1. Sit with a straight back.

2. Begin by observing the natural inhalation and exhalation of your breath without changing anything. If you find yourself distracted by the activity in your mind, try not to engage in the thoughts. Just notice them and then let them go, bringing your attention back to your inhalation and exhalation. Continue this for 30 to 60 seconds.

3. Now begin to breathe deeply through the nose. On each inhale, fill the belly with your breath. Expand the belly with air like a balloon. On each exhale, expel all the air out from the belly through your nose. Draw the navel back towards your spine to make sure that the belly is empty of air. Repeat this deep belly breathing for about five breaths.

4. On the next inhale, fill the belly up with air as described above. Then when the belly is full, draw in a little more breath and let that air expand into the rib cage causing the ribs to widen apart. On the exhale, let the air go first from the rib cage, letting the ribs slide closer together, and them from the belly, drawing the navel back towards the spine. Repeat this deep breathing into the belly and rib cage for about five breaths.

5. On the next inhale, fill the belly and rib cage with air as described above. Then draw in just a little more air and let it fill the upper chest, all the way up to the collarbone, causing the area around the heart (called the heart center in yoga) to expand and rise. On the exhale, let the breath go first from the upper chest, allowing the heart center to sink back down, then from the rib cage, letting the ribs slide closer together. Finally, let the air go from the belly, drawing the navel back towards the spine.

6. You are practicing three-part yogic breath! Continue at your own pace, eventually coming to let the three parts of the breath happen smoothly without pausing. Continue for about 10 breaths.

The great thing about this breathwork is that it can be done any-where—at home, in the car, at the office, at your kid's school while you are volunteering, during sporting events—anywhere! I like my patients to do 10 rounds 10 times a day. That gets your belly in the habit of relaxing. And guess what: If you can relax your belly, you cannot feel stressed. Try it. Try to be anxious with a soft belly. It's impossible.

Okay, so hopefully, you are beginning to understand how your thoughts activate your stress response system and how that then impacts genetic expression and the health of your gut and hormone system, which can then cause autoimmune disease. Now, let's get started on sorting the puzzle pieces and solving your puzzle.

Sorting the Pieces of the Puzzle

"Don't be satisfied with stories, how things have gone with others. Unfold your own myth."

~RUMI

Whenever I am putting a puzzle together, I look at the picture on the front of the box, which we have just done. Then I dump all the pieces out of the box onto a large table and begin sorting them. I want similar colors and patterns grouped on one part of the table. I want corner pieces separated from the center pieces. I find all of the edge pieces and then sort them into color and pattern groups. I want to make sure I have sorted the pieces as well as I can before I start snapping them together. It saves me a lot of time and frustration if I do a good job preparing the pieces before sitting down to put the puzzle together. Then, when I start putting the puzzle together, I do it just as methodically as I sorted it. I start by fitting the edge pieces together and into the corner pieces before I start filling in the interior.

When I help my patients solve their health puzzles, I am just as methodical. I use a combination of Ayurveda and Functional Medicine to sort out all of the pieces and organize all of the data.

Functional Medicine

Not long after making my Ayurveda-inspired lifestyle changes after my RA diagnosis, I discovered Functional Medicine. I realized this was a model that took the precepts of Ayurveda and translated them into Western language for the modern person in the Western world. Functional medicine, like Ayurvedic medicine, looks for the root cause of dis-ease rather than just managing the symptoms of disease. Functional medicine uses the latest scientific research to help you to understand yourself.

Both Functional and Ayurvedic medicine know that the root of wellness, as well as illness, is the digestive tract. Functional medicine provides in-depth testing and a way of sorting the data. Ayurvedic medicine's elegant framework of sorting individual body types and how they interact with the seasons, food, sleep, exercise, and life in general provides the ability to individualize care and treatment. This is integrative medicine. It's integrating the best of all worlds.

Functional and Ayurvedic medicine, or integrative medicine, empower you to take responsibility for your own health rather than turning yourself over to an "authority." This approach acknowledges that you are the first and last expert on you. This means you get the opportunity to understand that what you eat impacts how you digest and absorb nutrients. What you think impacts how you digest and absorb your experiences. Rather than focusing on an isolated set of symptoms, your integrative medicine provider will approach you as a whole person and create a relationship with you based on listening to your story and helping you find the clues, or puzzle pieces, so you can solve your puzzle.

Why See an Integrative Medicine Provider?

Functional medicine testing goes deeper than standard medical testing. Have you ever had the experience of going to your doctor, having some blood work done, and then being told you are fine—in spite of the fact that you feel terrible? Part of the problem is the insurance industry. Your insurance company only wants your medical provider to spend 6–10 minutes with you in a visit. This is not enough time to listen to your story, address the root problems of your symptoms, or to formulate a plan of action after educating you thoroughly about what's going on with your body. It's really only enough time to write you a prescription or order diagnostic tests.

Integrative medicine providers and health coaches spend time with their clients. They listen to their stories and evaluate the interactions among genetic, environmental, and lifestyle factors that can influence long-term health and complex, chronic imbalances. In this way, integrative medicine supports the unique expression of health and vitality for each individual.

Part of an integrative medicine approach to health is gathering the pieces of your unique puzzle. These are found in your story. You can map your story with the following exercise. Pay attention to what you learn about yourself. Are you able to make any connections? Do you learn anything new in this way of telling your story? This is valuable information to take to your next appointment with any integrative medicine provider or health coach.

Integration Exercise:
Creating Your Own Health Map

The solution to wandering around lost in the forest, or in the medical world, is to have a map. A map provides a way to see where you are, where you want to go, and how to get there. This Health Map is a key to freeing you from the "I don't know how I got sick" puzzle. It shows you that your current state of health did not happen "all of a sudden." It helps you track events from the past that are pieces to the puzzle of why you are feeling the way you are. It's based on a health tool the Institute for Functional Medicine uses for organizing information. I tweaked it a bit to fit with the Freedom Framework, which we will talk about next.

Instructions

1. Look at the Health Map tool (figure 7). By becoming aware of the state of your health story and where it is today, you will be able to rewrite it for the future. Your story begins with your conception. Do you know the story of your conception? If not, start from the earliest point of your life that you have information about. We start with conception and with prenatal care, because your vitality and health in utero are directly influenced by your mother's state of health and the health of your father's sperm. Ultimately, this impacts your health too.

2. Go through each of the four areas of energy on the left side bar to seek information: physical, mental, emotional, and spiritual. They all contribute to your current state of health.

3. Think about the story of your birth. What do you know? Go through each of the four areas of energy to seek information: physical, mental, emotional, and spiritual. They all contribute to your current state of health. Were your parents planning for you? Were you a surprise? Were you hard to conceive due to infertility issues? Was there a sibling who died before you were born? What were your parents' emotional states and levels of mental readiness at your birth? Were you born easily?

With the help of forceps? Vaginally or via a caesarian section (C-section)? Were you pink and vital when you arrived, or did it take a while to get you alert and warm? Did your mother receive anesthesia or have you naturally? At home or in the hospital? How long was her labor? Did she feel supported? Was your birth an epic story or rather uneventful? Tell your story here:

_____

_____

_____

_____

_____

_____

_____

_____

4. Next, look at the rest of the arrow (*see Figure 7 on page 67*) like a timeline and go through each of the four areas of energy to seek pieces to the puzzle of your health. Fill them in along the arrow in chronological order. Write in surgeries, illnesses, injuries, accidents, allergies, and food sensitivities. Don't forget about times you were on antibiotics, steroids, or other medications. Make sure you include any events from your emotional life such as past trauma, marriages, births, divorces, break-ups, and deaths. Include mental health and moods.

_____

_____

_____

_____

_____

_____

_____

_____

5. What are the elements of what I call your "period story," "libido story," and "menopause story?"

_____

_____

_____

_____

_____

_____

_____

_____

_____

6. When you are finished, take some time to explore your Health Map and write about your insights. What have you learned? What do you love about it? What would you like to rewrite? What meanings, beliefs, and behaviors did you create in childhood? Are any of them limiting you in your present life? If so, what would you like to replace these outdated beliefs with in terms of powerful meanings, beliefs, and life-sustaining behaviors? What action can you take today that might shift a self-limiting behavior tomorrow?

_____

_____

_____

_____

_____

_____

_____

_____

_____

7. What would it look like for you to have perfect health? What would "good enough" health look like? What are your goals for your health?

What would you be able to be and do in your life if you, your mind, your body, and your heart were all on the same page and aligned?

_____

_____

_____

_____

_____

_____

_____

_____

8. Write what you are willing to shift in your life to attain your goals. Now that you see your Health Map drawn out, what do you need to change to attain the level of vitality you really desire?

_____

_____

_____

_____

_____

_____

_____

_____

9. Now that you have completed this exercise, what is one healthy habit you can commit to adopting today that will improve your quality of life? Remember that the first 30 seconds of any new habit are the most important ones. Those first 30 seconds are moving you into the first minute of a new healthy habit. That first minute is the first of the next 30 minutes. Those first 30 minutes are the first minutes of the next 24 hours. No matter what, 24 hours are going to pass for you. It is up to you how you choose to spend them. I encourage you to take that first 30 second step to a powerful new way of being!

_____

_____

_____

_____

_____

_____

_____

_____

_____

_____

▼ **Figure 7**

Health Map Worksheet

(adapted from the Institute for Functional Medicine's Timeline)

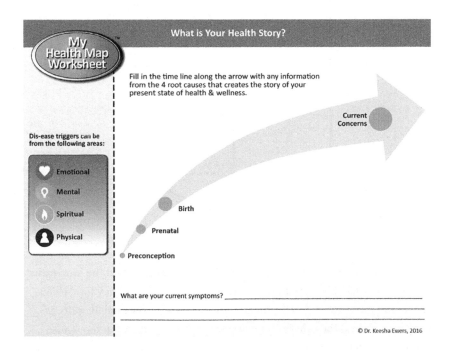

How to Solve the Autoimmune Puzzle

A New Perspective

Have you ever looked at a Necker Cube? The Necker cube, first published in 1832 by Louise Albert Necker, is a simple way of demonstrating the power of perception and perspective. Take a look at the cube in the *Figure 8*. Like most people who view it for the first time, do you notice the left lower corner pointing out? Now stare at a different part of the cube (especially try staring at the center rectangle). Do you notice the perspective shift? Can you see the right upper corner pointing out now? You might need to soften your gaze, glance away from the cube and come back, or close your eyes and open them again to get the cube to shift.

▼ **Figure 8**

The Necker Cube

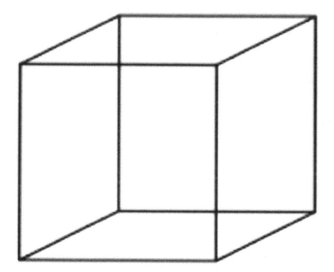

This is much like the Uncle SAM model of healthcare and the integrative medicine model. They are both models of healthcare, but they have different dominant features and perspectives. One is based on matching drugs to symptoms and the other is based on solving the issue at the root cause. Both are models, just as the cube above is just a cube. How you see the cube is just a matter of perspective, and now that you know the secret, how you want to see it. You can train your brain to see it differently if you want to.

I am going to teach you a different way to see your symptoms. It's a new perspective. It's how you will sort the smaller puzzle pieces of your health puzzle from now on. This method freed me from my own illness, thought patterns, emotional ups and downs, self-sabotaging beliefs and behaviors, and helped me create a life I am in love with. That's why I call it the Freedom Framework. It's the frame to your puzzle, the outside edges that all of the smaller pieces snap into. It's one more sorting tool that we are going to use to help you solve your puzzle.

The Freedom Framework

I look at the Uncle SAM model of healthcare as being "in the matrix," and functional or integrative or Ayurvedic medicine as being "outside of the matrix." Like the blockbuster movie, *The Matrix*, the people in the matrix are living in a system that says it's taking care of them. The people in the matrix don't know that this isn't the case. They believe that if Uncle SAM's Food and Drug Administration (FDA) passes a drug, it's safe. They believe that if the government allows genetically modified organisms (GMO), or foods on the shelves in our grocery stores, they must be safe. They believe doctors trained in the matrix who say, "Diet has nothing to do with what is happening to you or why you have this disease." As I mentioned earlier, the miracles of modern medicine should not be overlooked. There is no better place to be if you have a heart attack, break your arm, or are in a car accident. The "miracle of modern medicine" is not, however, for preventing disease or reversing autoimmunity.

Once outside of the matrix, you are free, but also responsible for keeping yourself healthy. It's a harder world when you take full responsibility for what you put on your fork or in your glass. You can no longer turn a blind eye when you are outside of the matrix. You know your choices influence your quality of life. The Freedom Framework takes you out of the matrix and sets you free of the "one-size-fits-all" mentality. This is where you learn to prevent disease and to optimize your energy and health so you can live your life purpose.

Once again, the four pillars of the Freedom Framework are:

1. un-**C**over root cause(s).
2. **C**onfront the data collected through laboratory testing and your story.
3. **C**onnect your beliefs and behaviors with your current reality.
4. **C**reate the life you want to be living with full intention.

Let's start with the beginning, un-Cover root causes.

Un-Cover Root Cause(s)

There are five root causes to every kind of dis-ease, including autoimmune diseases. By searching through each of these five root causes, you will find the solution to your puzzle 100% of the time, guaranteed. The five root causes are:

1. Physical
2. Mental
3. Emotional
4. Spiritual
5. Your Story

You will find as we work with the Freedom Framework that these will often overlap. You are not separate body systems, you are a whole being.

Physical

The first root cause is the body. I start with the body because the body holds the record of your past hurts, traumas, cognitive distortions, and lifestyle choices. It also contains the impact of your exposure to toxins, your ability to detox those toxicants, and the impact your life experiences to date have had on your genetic expression. Your body is the repository of all you have experienced and has a lot to tell you in terms of how well it's doing. The question is, are you listening?

When you are scanning the body for possible causes for your autoimmune disease, you will want to do comprehensive functional medicine laboratory testing (Chapter 9). Always test rather than guess at what is going on in the body. You will also want to learn the body's elegant and simple language it uses to communicate with you (Chapter 10). Your pain level, your menstrual cycle, your skin, tongue, eyes, energy and libido levels, weight, measurements, body odor, bowel movement, fingernails, facial lines, and urine are all ways your body is keeping you apprised of how it's doing.

If you are a diabetic, you monitor your blood-sugar level, insulin level, and Hgb A1c. If you have high blood pressure, you monitor your blood pressure. If you wear glasses, you get your eyes checked. These monitoring tools are done for diseases that are already active. Your body has quieter ways of talking to you before it's in a disease state. I am going to teach you to tune in so it no longer has to crank the volume up to get your attention.

Mental

The second root cause is the mind. Why? Because your perceptions of stress are what activate your 4F stress response, get out of danger, response system. Mind-body medicine is a term used to illustrate that what happens in the body has a direct correlation with what is going on in the mind. On my own journey out of autoimmune disease, I discovered that a rigid mind creates a rigid body. This is why I call the relationship between your mind and the autoimmune process occurring in your body the autoimmune mindset.

Remember the four corners of the autoimmune puzzle? They are genetics, toxins, leaky gut, and trauma. Toxins are not just the environmental kind, such as pesticides, pollutants, and other estrogen-disrupting chemicals. They are also the mental kind. Toxic thoughts create toxic beliefs and self-sabotaging behaviors and habits. Examples of toxic thoughts are:

"I'm unlovable."

"I'm not deserving of _____ (love, money, safety, friendships, God, etc.)."

"I'm not good enough."

"I'm too fat."

"I'm broken."

"I'm sick."

"I'm bad."

"He's bad." or "She's bad."

"At least I'm better than her/him."

"I have to be perfect."

"I am perfect."

"God loves me more than He/She loves ____."

"He/She deserves what he/she gets."

"I'm not safe."

"Life is too hard."

"Nothing ever goes my way."

"Nobody understands me."

"I have never had a happy moment in life."

"Life isn't fair."

"Why am I the only one who is suffering?"

"If I am nice, others will be nice to me."

"If I am fair, others will treat me fairly."

"If my mother/father/husband/wife/sibling/child/God really loved me, she/he would know what I need."

"I need to make everyone happy."

"If I lose ___ pounds, or make ____ dollars, or get to vacation in ____, or buy this ____, I will be happy."

This list contains examples of what are called cognitive distortions. This list is by no means complete. It contains a few examples of beliefs that, when held onto, will cause suffering. Where do these beliefs come from? They were created in childhood as a way of making meaning from life experiences. The irony about distorted beliefs is they are created by child brains, which means undeveloped brains.

The Trouble with Undeveloped Brains

The brain is not fully developed until you are about 26 years of age. The frontal cortex is still developing throughout childhood and young adulthood. This is the part of the brain in charge of judgment, decision-making, and impulse control. Notice the first two I listed—judgment and decision-making. You were judging your experiences in childhood, or making up meanings to make sense of them, without a fully developed brain.

We sort out the information we take in and then compare it for context and meaning against memories of earlier experiences and meanings. But what happens when you are taking in data for the very first time? When you are a child, you are experiencing events that you have never had before. It's like fresh snow. There are no footprints or tire tracks yet. What happens if there is no wise adult at hand to help you make sense of this fresh new information? When it's your first snow, there is a bit of magic and wonder that you might record in your memory vault, even without the help of a wise and attuned adult.

But what if it's not a wonderful event you are experiencing? What if you just watched your dad hit your mother? What if you are crying in your crib hour after hour with a wet diaper and a hungry belly and your caregiver is too drunk or high to meet your needs? What if you moved to a new school leaving your friends behind, and the new kids don't seem to like you? What if your parents get divorced? How about failing a test at school, not making the team, getting left off the invitation list for a birthday party? What do you do with sexual abuse from someone you trust when you haven't even learned what the word sex means and don't understand what abuse is?

The answer to the above questions is…you make sh*t up. That's right. You create a story and make up a meaning to fit what you just experienced. The meanings you created to help you understand your life events from your early years were then hardwired into your system as a survival strategy. They helped form your personality and are what you now call your beliefs or world view. Those beliefs then led to the actions you took to navigate the unchartered waters of your youth. Your meanings and beliefs formed your decisions about how to behave, which then crystalized into habits if you felt that you got your needs met adequately.

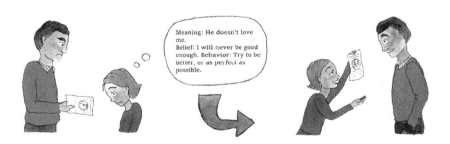

▲ *Undeveloped brain making up a story*

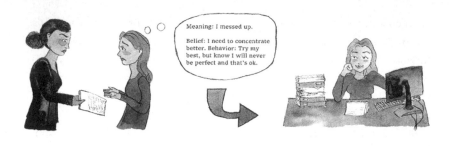

▲ *Developed brain able to use upset as feedback for improvement*

Now most of your beliefs, behaviors, and habits were formed in child-hood—again, with a brain that was not yet fully developed. Further, they were often created in times of uncertainty and even crisis or trauma. It's like giving a four-year-old the keys to your car and expecting her to do a good job driving. Four-year-old children can't even see over the dashboard, let alone get you to where you need to go. Do you want the meanings, beliefs, and behaviors that came from an undeveloped brain to be your present-day operating system? Maybe it's time for an upgrade. You do this when your computer is outdated, why not upgrade your belief system to match your current level of brain development? I will take you through a process for doing this in Chapter 11.

Emotional

In Chapter 11 you will learn how the heart holds onto unresolved hurt. We all experience emotional pain in life; it's part of the human experience. How that hurt influences your future relationships, your quality of life, and your willingness to forgive and set healthy boundaries, depends upon the context of the hurt, your developmental stage, and the story you tell after-wards. The more you tell your story from a victim's perspective, the more deeply ingrained it becomes in your body.

Remember, rigid mind=rigid body. All children are powerless. Think back to your childhood. You were told what to eat, how to dress, how to artic-ulate, how to treat others, how to view the world and those you share the planet with, and much more. Every child is victimized many times during their development. Again, this is part of life. As you will learn later, the degree of victimization makes a huge difference in how your brain develops, what your state of health is in adulthood, and how willing you are to care for yourself.

Healing un-resolved trauma (HURT) from your past is essential if you are going to reverse autoimmunity, or better yet, prevent it. If you hold onto your emotional pain in your body, it will create what we'll call a "button." That button can then be pushed by people you relate with for the rest of your life. Harboring fear of future hurt is what causes many people to wall off their hearts and face the world with the protection of their ego selves. We will talk more about this later. I am going to teach you a process for moving emotional hurt and pain out of your body, for forgiving for your own sake, and for setting good boundaries with toxic people, toxic foods and drinks, and toxic beliefs. I will help you to understand the difference between unskillful ways of feeling powerful in your life and skillful ways of *being* powerful.

Spiritual

The fourth root cause of dis-ease is spirituality, spirit, and energy. Spirit and energy are often used interchangeably by people who have varying views of what spirit means. The spiritual or religious tradition you were raised in will impact your adult health. Think about it. If you were taught that having enough faith that God will heal you, and you feel chronically sick, do you then judge yourself as unfaithful? What did your religious tradition say about the unfaithful? Did they inherit the Kingdom of Heaven? Again, unexamined childhood beliefs can become pain in the adult body. Do you believe yourself abandoned by God? Betrayed by God? Being punished by God?

People who consider themselves spiritual, rather than religious, have their own relationship with spirit, sometimes referencing this as Source, the Divine, or simply energy.

The World of Energy

When I say energy, I am going beyond what you might typically call energy. I don't mean the energy it takes to go to the gym or how many tasks from your list of things to do you can accomplish in a day. I am talking about your energy *body*. This is the layer of the body called prana in Ayurveda, chi in Chinese medicine, and ki in Japanese (as in Reiki). Energy is what the world is made of. Energy is what enlivens all that is living. Everything has energy. Everything is energy. I look at spirit in the same way I look at energy. In Eastern philosophy, the primordial force of energy thought to create and move through the entire Universe is called Shakti. Any dis-ease that you can think of will include an energy block somewhere in your physical, mental, or emotional being. This will profoundly affect your connection to spirit.

The energetic body responds to the energy you put into it. You might have heard this said as, "garbage in, garbage out." If you eat foods low in life force, such as anything coming from a can, package, or box, you will not feel as energized as you would if you drank a glass full of freshly juiced vegetables. If you go to sleep after watching 30 minutes of depressing news commentary about how the planet and the people who inhabit it are self-combusting, you will not awaken as refreshed as you would if you took a lovely salt bath, followed by a self-massage with warm sesame oil just before bed. Binge watching anything on television will not bring you the same energetic response from your body, mind, and heart as getting outdoors in nature will. Think about how you feel after spending time with someone who is toxic versus someone who encourages and supports you in being the best version of yourself that you can be. Later, I will give you some tools for clearing your energy body as a way of reversing autoimmunity.

Story

The elements of your story and how you tell it is the last root cause in this first pillar of the Freedom Framework. You are the hero and the creator of your own story. Think for a moment about what kind of story you are living right this minute in your life. Is it a fast-paced action drama? Is it a horror story? A tragedy? A romance? A comedy?

What role do you play in this story? Are you a brave and courageous hero, willing to take on whatever life hands you? Are you a damsel in distress waiting to be rescued from an unhappy life? Are you a victim, a martyr, an emotional vampire, a jester, a peacemaker, a rescuer, a hermit, a skeptic, a seeker, a sage, a student, a teacher, a maiden, a matron, or a matriarch? Are you a princess or a tyrant? Are you an orphan, feeling abandoned, or are you a bully beating up on those weaker than you? What genre of story would you like to be living? What role do you want to play in it? Are you living the story you want to live?

It's likely that your life story to this point is a mix of many of the genres I have mentioned and you have played many roles. However, you might have a little too much of one kind that is making you unhappy. You might feel stuck in a story you never thought you would be in, playing a part you don't want to play any longer. I know that the way I tell my story is much different today than I did 20 years ago when I had autoimmunity. I now look at my distressing childhood experiences and even my autoimmune disease as gifts that helped me to grow and become who I am today. You will learn an exercise that will teach you to re-frame your thoughts if you are feeling like a victim of circumstances beyond your control (Chapter 12).

Let's move on to the second part of the puzzle frame, or Freedom Framework: Confronting the Data you collected in Step One.

Confronting the Data

You can't change what you haven't realized, and you can't realize what you haven't confronted.

Confronting the data is the second part of the frame to your puzzle, which is to say, it's the second pillar of the Freedom Framework. This means you self-confront, you confront the data you have received from your laboratory work. You confront the root causes that have just been uncovered in the first pillar. I call this truth-telling time. It's time to get very clear about what is going on with you, in all your layers.

Connecting the Dots

Connecting the dots means connecting your lifestyle choices, your beliefs, and your behaviors to the reality you are living today. This is the third side of your puzzle frame, the third pillar of the Freedom Framework. This step brings Isaac Newton's third law of motion home: For every action, there is an equal and opposite reaction. This is why a pill will not solve the root cause of your weight, fatigue, or pain. Being willing to connect your behaviors to your reality means you take care of the causes you find at the root of your problem.

When a plant is wilting, you don't paint the leaves green. Hopefully you stick your finger in the soil to see if it's dry, check out how much light it's getting, look at the leaves to see if there are bugs that don't belong there, investigate the soil for mold and rot, and look to see if the plant has outgrown its pot. This is exactly what I do with my patients. I look at data points and then help them make the connections. The Uncle SAM model of healthcare paints the leaves of the wilted plant green. This is not a sustainable solution for your health.

You will be introduced to the HURT Model in Chapter 10. HURT stands for **H**ealing **u**n-**r**esolved **t**rauma. This model shows where you have a choice point when you are confronted with any stressful situation. You can choose to act or choose to react. Re-acting means you have had this same action or behavior in the past; now it's a RE-action. You are repeating a pattern of action in response to a trigger that was created in childhood.

Acting proactively will mean you are behaving in a new, more powerful way. This will result in a more powerful outcome. Reacting in negative patterns of behavior can keep you stuck in disease. *Creating adaptive behaviors that are a result of powerful beliefs and meanings can set you free from disease.*

Reactive behavior lacks the ability to self-confront. If your reactive mind and immune system stay set at default settings, then you will remain sick. Proactive behavior requires self-confrontation. It requires pause and examination of perceptions, meanings, and beliefs. It takes some courage to drop into self-inquiry to find out if what you are perceiving is real. You then have an opportunity to build a new skill that will result in freedom from a hyper-vigilant immune system, or autoimmunity.

Create the Life You Desire with Intention

The fourth side of your puzzle is the fourth pillar of the Freedom Framework. Step four is about getting powerfully intentional about creating the life you want to be living. What is the body you want to live in? What are you willing to do to get it? Negotiate your priorities. Navigate your schedule. Be willing to ruthlessly cut out beliefs, behaviors, activities, foods, and people who do not support the highest and best potential for your life.

I will be giving you some integration exercises to help you move from the passive, default settings your meanings created in childhood, to upgraded, intentional-living settings. Finally, remember that growth is not linear. It's a spiral, like a labyrinth. Be willing to circle back again on the same patterns you think you have already dealt with, but this time at a deeper level. You will always be mining the same areas of your psyche for the obstacles to your freedom (so you can release them) as you work with the fourth "missing piece" of the autoimmune puzzle—past trauma.

How many wonderful podcasts, talks, or sermons have you heard that have lifted you up and brought you new awareness? How many self-help books, articles, or blogs have you read that have given you "ah-ha" moments? How many classes, workshops, or webinars have you taken, only to come home and find that you slip back into your default ways of being?

Why do you revert back to default settings? I believe it's because your default settings were set up in the factory—otherwise known as your family of origin or childhood home—and encrypted by your ego so they would be difficult to hack. Apple phones are not as hard to get into as your subconscious default settings are, I assure you. As you age and grow, your hardware is changing and updating. But if you are not consciously rewriting software to keep up with the needs for updates, you are going to find yourself crashing constantly.

So how do you make those updates? Well, you need an encryption key to hack your system. The best one I have found is provided by functional medicine. It's called the 5 R's of healing.

The 5 R's of Healing
(the center pieces to your puzzle)

We live in an instant gratification society that likes to focus on quick fixes and magic pills. We are all incredibly busy with tight schedules. However, the magic pill theory simply doesn't work. Why do I say that? In spite of spending million—no, billions—of dollars on healthcare, research, and drug development, the numbers of women (and men and children) being diagnosed with autoimmune disease continue to escalate. There is no magic pill, no magic wand, and no magic diet.

Functional medicine focuses on getting to the root cause of illness. It's a great alternative to the Uncle SAM model of healthcare. The 5 R's of functional medicine will help you put your puzzle together and ultimately help you heal the root causes of your autoimmunity (*see figure 9*). They are:

1. **R**emove
2. **R**eplace
3. **R**epair
4. **R**e-inoculate
5. **R**ebalance

The 5 R's of healing autoimmune disease

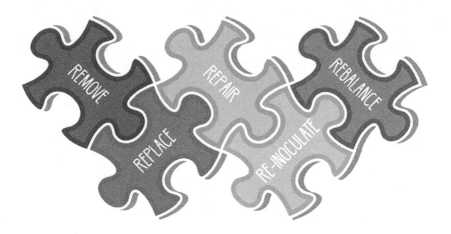

The meaning of these and how to apply them to your personal situation is best discovered through your own experience, which is just what you will have the chance to do in the following exercise. Writing allows you to release stored thoughts and reactions that might be chaotic jumble in your mind. The act of writing helps to create order out of chaos. Enjoy the process and take your time.

Integration Exercise: Patterns of Reaction

Again, you have default settings of reactivity that you set up in childhood through the meanings you made up to explain the experiences of your childhood. Some of those experiences were difficult, others happy. Understanding what sets off your 4F response system is a great first step to re-wire it, to reduce its sensitivity. That's what this exercise is for.

1. Think about what makes you angry. When was the last time you got angry? Maybe you don't believe you get angry. In that case, when was

the last time you were frustrated, annoyed, irritated, or impatient? What caused it? Write your triggers here:

_____

_____

_____

_____

_____

_____

_____

_____

2. Next, write how you respond to the events that trigger you. When you are angry, how would I know you are angry? Does your face flush? Do you clench your jaw? Do you get knots in your tummy? Do you stop breathing? Do you withdraw? Do you shout? Do you say things you regret later? Do you lash out physically? Do you melt down emotionally? Write this down.

_____

_____

_____

_____

_____

_____

_____

3. Think about how this pattern serves you. What do you get from it? Does it make people stop the offending behavior? Does it help you feel safe? Does it annoy the person who has irritated you? Does it make you feel powerless or powerful? Write this down.

_____

_____

_____

_____

_____

_____

_____

_____

_____

_____

4. Now think about how your pattern doesn't serve you. Is it an outdated response mode? How old were you when you started this pattern? Do you remember why you began coping in this way? Do you feel trapped by your outdated default setting? Do you need a software upgrade? Is it time to reprogram your system? You can change your final puzzle picture by confronting these patterns. Write down your impressions:

_____

_____

_____

_____

_____

_____

_____

_____

Think of this exercise as an opportunity to change the center pieces of your puzzle. If you find outdated patterns, you get to shift them using the 5 R's: 1) **R**emove, 2) **R**eplace, 3) **R**epair, 4) **R**e-inoculate, and 5) **R**ebalance.

Fill in the blanks below with what from the above exercise you would like to **R**emove. What is a more powerful way you could respond to your typical triggers and upsets? (In other words, what will you **R**eplace those patterns with?) What part of your childhood meaning needs to be **R**epaired? What is a powerful affirmation you can use to **R**e-inoculate your psyche with? Finally, how do you need to **R**ebalance? A rigid mind will create a rigid body. What are the action steps you can begin immediately that will start softening your nervous system's reactive response?

1. **Remove:**

_____

_____

_____

_____

2. **Remove:**

_____

_____

_____

_____

3. **Repair:**

_____

_____

_____

_____

4. **Re-inoculate:**

_____

_____

_____

_____

5. **Rebalance:**

_____

_____

_____

_____

Congratulations! You are on the path to reversing your autoimmune disease.

SECTION II:
The Cornerstone Pieces of the Autoimmune Puzzle

"The most effective way to do it, is to do it."

~AMELIA EARHART

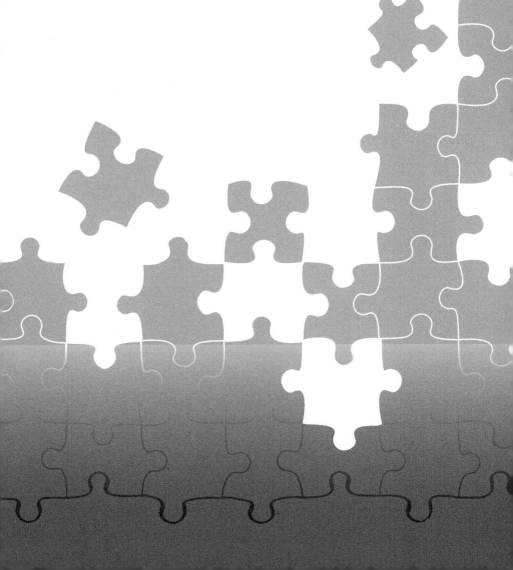

Sorting the Pieces of the Puzzle

"Our sorrows and wounds are healed only when we touch them with compassion."

~BUDDHA

The Missing Piece of the Autoimmune Puzzle

Now that you have seen the big picture, been introduced to the pieces of the puzzle, learned how to frame your puzzle and how to change the middle pieces by using the 5 R's, it's time to spend some time on the four corner pieces. What are the four corner pieces? The root causes of autoimmune disease: childhood trauma, genetics, toxins, and leaky gut.

I call childhood trauma the missing piece of the autoimmune puzzle. The other three pieces are now widely known thanks to the pioneering work of Dr. Alessio Fassano. Fassano identified three root causes to autoimmune disease: genetics, environmental toxins, and leaky gut. Most functional medicine providers are aware of these root causes and focus on them in their protocols. Yet women are still falling through the cracks and getting frustrated. Focus on the three root causes is good, but it's not enough.

In my practice, I see time and again that supplements and diets are not ending autoimmunity in women. On a daily basis, I see angry women who follow these protocols prescribed by their doctors, believe they are "doing everything right" with their diets, take the supplements they have been ordered, and yet feel that the ice they are standing on is melting as their diets get more and more restricted and good health eludes them. I recently had a woman in my office who cried as she told me she was down to eating only five foods. "My world is shrinking," she sobbed.

Naturally, when we talk about leaky gut, genetics, and environmental toxins, we talk about stress. However, it is in a rather off-handed way. It's not getting to the core of *why* women hold onto their immune reactivity. The immune system will mirror the mental system. If the mind is reactive, the immune system will follow. Is there any science to prove this? Yes. There are several studies, but I am going to focus on one in particular: the ACE (Adverse Childhood Experiences) study.

The ACE Study

The Adverse Childhood Experiences Study (ACE Study) was conducted by the Centers for Disease Control and Prevention (CDC) and Kaiser Permanente between 1995 and 1997.

In the 1980s, in spite of the fact that the participants at Kaiser Permanente's obesity clinic were all successfully losing weight, about 50% were dropping out. This was confusing to the founder of the Department of Preventive Medicine for Kaiser Permanente, Vincent Felitti. Dr. Felitti interviewed many of the people who had left the program and discovered that a majority of the 286 people he interviewed had experienced childhood sexual abuse. These conversations revealed to Felitti that weight gain could be less about food and hunger and more about coping with depression, anxiety, and fear.

Dr. Robert Anda of the CDC joined Felitti and went on to survey childhood trauma experiences of over 17,000 Kaiser Permanente patient volunteers. Of the 17,337 study participants, half were female. (Three-fourths of the total were white with an average age of 57 and college educated.) All had jobs and good healthcare. They were asked about distressing childhood experiences, including abuse and neglect.

The 10 items that were covered were:
1. Physical abuse
2. Sexual abuse
3. Emotional abuse
4. Physical neglect
5. Emotional neglect
6. Mother was treated violently
7. Household substance abuse

8. Household mental illness
9. Parental separation or divorce
10. Incarcerated household member

If one of the 10 items applied to a participant, it counted as a "1," or an ACE score of "1." If a participant reported 2 adverse events, she had an ACE score of "2," and so on.

ACE Study Findings

Dr. Felitti is reported to have broken down and wept when he saw the results of the survey. Over 2/3 of the study participants reported an ACE score of one or more. Of these, 87% reported at least one more ACE. A staggering 40% of the participants reported two or more ACEs, and 12.5% experienced four or more. Some participants experienced divorced parents or had an absent or addictive caregiver. Twenty-eight percent were physically abused and 21% sexually abused (*see figure 10*).

▼ **Figure 10**

Examples of abuse and neglect

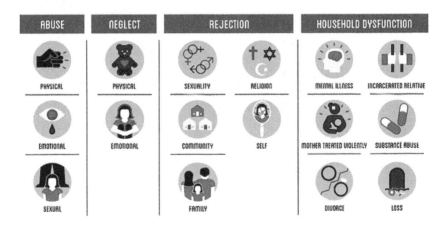

Compared to an ACE score of zero, having four or more ACEs creates a seven-fold increase in alcoholism, doubles the risk of cancer, and quadruples the incidence of emphysema. An ACE score over six creates a 30-fold increase in attempted suicide (*see figure 11*).

▼ **Figure 11**

Risk factors of ACEs

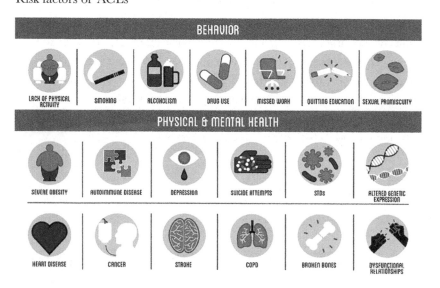

The study found that the higher the ACE score, the higher the risk for developing chronic disease and other health-related issues: autoimmune disease, heart disease, cancer, diabetes, depression, addiction(s), suicide, social issues, high-risk health behaviors, obesity, and behavioral problems (*see figure 12*). In other words, what happened in their childhood continued to have an impact into adulthood and throughout the shortened life spans of these initial volunteers. Indeed, the ACE study's results indicate that mistreatment and household dysfunction in the early years contribute to the most common causes of death and disability decades later. A further shocking finding of this study: adverse childhood experiences are all too common. (This has been verified in subsequent studies using different screening tools.)

▼ Figure 12

The higher the ACEs, the higher the risk for autoimmune (and other chronic) disease

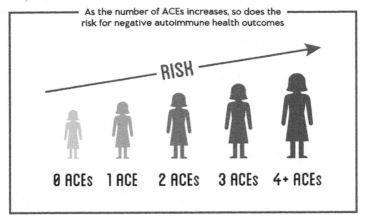

The ACE Quiz

An ACE score is the total of 10 different types of abuse, neglect, and household dysfunction. The ACE quiz is by no means exhaustive, with the glaring absence of death and loss. However, it does correlate early distressing events from childhood with adult chronic illness like autoimmune disease. According to the Adverse Childhood Experiences study, the tougher your childhood, the higher your score is likely to be, and the higher your risk for later chronic disease and even a shortened life span (*see figure 13*).

▼ Figure 13

The higher the ACEs, the lower the life span

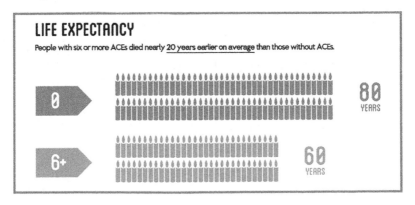

Here is the test, if you would like to know your own ACE score.

1. Before your 18th birthday, did a parent or other adult in the household often or very often...swear at you, insult you, put you down, or humiliate you? or act in a way that made you afraid that you might be physically hurt?

    YES / NO

2. Before your 18th birthday, did a parent or other adult in the household often or very often...push, grab, slap, or throw something at you? or ever hit/spank you so hard that you had marks or were injured?

    YES / NO

3. Before your 18th birthday, did an adult or person at least five years older than you ever...touch or fondle you or have you touch their body in a sexual way? or attempt or actually have oral, anal, or vaginal intercourse with you?

    YES / NO

4. Before your eighteenth birthday, did you often or very often feel that...no one in your family loved you or thought you were important or special? or your family didn't look out for each other, feel close to each other, or support each other?

    YES / NO

5. Before your 18th birthday, did you often or very often feel that... you didn't have enough to eat, had to wear dirty clothes, and had no one to protect you? or your parents were too drunk or high to take care of you or take you to the doctor if you needed it?

    YES / NO

6. Before your 18th birthday, was a biological parent ever lost to you through divorce, abandonment, or other reason?

YES / NO

7. Before your 18th birthday, was your mother or stepmother: often or very often pushed, grabbed, slapped, or had something thrown at her? or sometimes, often, or very often kicked, bitten, hit with a fist, or hit with something hard? or ever repeatedly hit over at least a few minutes or threatened with a gun or knife?

YES / NO

8. Before your 18th birthday, did you live with anyone who was a problem drinker or alcoholic, or who used street drugs?

YES / NO

9. Before your 18th birthday, was a household member depressed or mentally ill, or did a household member attempt suicide?

YES / NO

10. Before your 18th birthday, did a household member go to prison?

YES / NO

Some ACE Definitions

ABUSE

Emotional abuse: A parent, stepparent, or adult living in your home swore at you, insulted you, put you down, or acted in a way that made you afraid that you might be physically hurt.

Physical abuse: A parent, stepparent, or adult living in your home pushed, grabbed, slapped, threw something at you, or hit you so hard that you had marks or were injured.

Sexual abuse: An adult, relative, family friend, or stranger who was at least 5 years older than you ever touched or fondled your body in a sexual way, made you touch his/her body in a sexual way, attempted to have any type of sexual intercourse with you.

HOUSEHOLD CHALLENGES

Mother treated violently: Your mother or stepmother was pushed, grabbed, slapped, had something thrown at her, kicked, bitten, hit with a fist, hit with something hard, repeatedly hit for over at least a few minutes, or ever threatened or hurt by a knife or gun by your father (or stepfather) or mother's boyfriend.

Household substance abuse: A household member was a problem drinker or alcoholic or a household member used street drugs.

Mental illness in household: A household member was depressed or mentally ill or a household member attempted suicide.

Parental separation or divorce: Your parents were ever separated or divorced.

Criminal household member: A household member went to prison.

NEGLECT

Emotional neglect: Someone in your family helped you feel important or special, you felt loved, people in your family looked out for each other and felt close to each other, and your family was a source of strength and support.[1]

Physical neglect: There was someone to take care of you, protect you, and take you to the doctor if you needed it, [1]you didn't have enough to eat, your parents were too drunk or too high to take care of you, and you had to wear dirty clothes.

---

[1] Items were reverse-scored to reflect the framing of the question.

Your ACE Score Impacts Your Level of Self-Care

Self-neglect is a pattern I see in a lot of women with autoimmune disease. I certainly was guilty of it myself. When I say self-neglect, I am again referring to taking time for real self-care. I exercised every day (to an extreme), took a shower, dressed nicely, ate three meals a day, etc. However, I did not put myself at the top of the list for making sure I had enough quiet time for self-inquiry. Self-inquiry and self-confrontation are what build self-awareness. Self-awareness leads to the ability to progress developmentally and lowers emotional and mental reactivity. Remember that a rigid mind leads to a rigid body and immune system. Or another way I like to say this, "What's in your head goes to your bed." Check in with yourself and make sure you are spending plenty of time each day in self-inquiry. It will allow you to break free of patterns such as emotional over-eating, self-sabotaging behaviors, and outright self-neglect (*see figure 14*).

You Have Your ACE Score. What Next?

First of all, the ACE score is meant to be helpful, not to freak you out. Secondly, as you will see in this book, early childhood distress is one of several pieces to your health puzzle. It snaps in as a corner piece and joins your genetics, toxic exposure, and leaky gut to the autoimmune framework. We are putting this puzzle together a piece at a time, and doing it together. I am going to show you that your ACE score does not set your future in stone, any more than your DNA does. The mission of this book is to provide you with a method for altering each of your puzzle pieces until your health picture is just how you want it to be.

So, hang onto that ACE score and read on. You are going to discover how to reverse the impact your early childhood events have had on your current health puzzle. One of the pieces the ACE quiz doesn't ask about is your positive early life experiences. These are what help you build resilience and protect you from the impact of the distressing events every person has in life.

Positive experiences are provided through relationships with good teachers, loving grandparents, a friend who believes in you, a great therapist, a compassionate spiritual leader, a connection to your spiritual beliefs, or an attuned parent. You are going to learn simple resilience-building tools in the next few chapters. You are going to learn how to become the attuned caregiver for yourself that you have always needed and perhaps been trying to

▼ **Figure 14**

Patterns of Self-Neglect

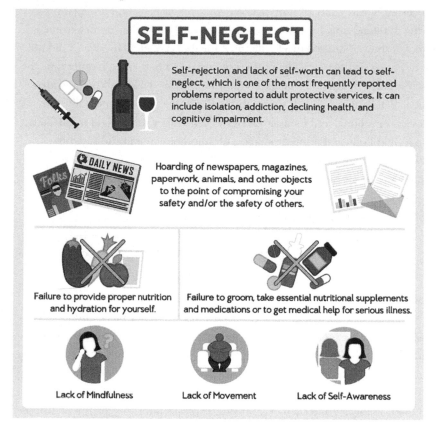

SELF-NEGLECT

Self-rejection and lack of self-worth can lead to self-neglect, which is one of the most frequently reported problems reported to adult protective services. It can include isolation, addiction, declining health, and cognitive impairment.

Hoarding of newspapers, magazines, paperwork, animals, and other objects to the point of compromising your safety and/or the safety of others.

Failure to provide proper nutrition and hydration for yourself.

Failure to groom, take essential nutritional supplements and medications or to get medical help for serious illness.

Lack of Mindfulness

Lack of Movement

Lack of Self-Awareness

find unsuccessfully in others. Again, the ability to change your brain, express your genetics in a healthy way, and to detox old hurts takes *willingness*. Willingness is the first and most important quality to cultivate in yourself as you learn to reverse your autoimmunity and inflammation.

In each of the next few chapters, I will introduce you to four patients of mine who have had their names and some details of their stories altered. They each have four things in common: 1) they are female, 2) they had autoimmune disease, 3) they were willing to make the life changes necessary to reverse their autoimmunity, and 4) they all reversed their diseases. You will notice that they all had events or lifestyle choices that fall into all four of the root causes for autoimmune disease: toxins, genetics, leaky gut, and trauma.

Dr. Tom O'Bryan talks about the autoimmune spectrum. How many factors you have in your life from those four cornerstone root causes will influence where you fall on the autoimmune spectrum. If you have mild inflammation and very few symptoms, or what I call low misery, you will be on one side of the spectrum. If you have developed three autoimmune diseases and are severely miserable, you are on the other side of the autoimmune spectrum.

I call this critical mass (*see figure 15*). The more hits to your immune system, the heavier the load and the more likely your boat will capsize. Each of the patients I am introducing you to were capsized due to critical mass. They were all miserable when they came to see me and all very motivated to make the changes that lightened the load so they could float once again.

▼ Figure 15

Critical mass will capsize your health and vitality

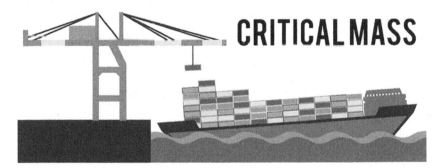

Let's begin with Mica.

Mica

When Mica came to see me, it was for a self-diagnosed hormone imbalance. She was having hot flashes and insomnia and struggling with fatigue. I noticed she was wearing a loose caftan and flip flops and her arms were covered with red, angry welts. When I commented on them, she nodded her head and grimly told me that the state of her skin at that moment was about 50% better than it had been the week before. She told me briefly about how this outbreak had occurred.

She had just returned home from visiting a family member who used commercial detergent on the bed linens. It only took one night in the bed and she was inflamed, fatigued, itchy, and unable to sleep for the rest of her stay. She then tried to re-direct me back to her "hormone issues," telling me that she had the whole skin thing controlled with prescription steroids and over-the-counter antihistamines. I let her know that her hormones and her skin were very much related. She looked surprised, but was open to hearing what I had to say.

When I asked Mica to tell me her history, I found many pieces to her puzzle. She clearly had autoimmune disease, but didn't know it. Her immune system was amped up and attacking friendly cells as well as the foreign invaders she was exposed to. It turned out Mica would break out at the slightest provocation. She found it difficult to travel, to eat, and had to be very careful with the fabrics and products that touched her skin. Her bubble of tolerance was shrinking the older she got.

I used the Freedom Framework to organize Mica's puzzle pieces. I paid careful attention to her story and to the language she used to tell it. I asked about her physical health, mental health, emotional health, and spiritual health to tease out the root causes of her autoimmune disease.

Step One: Un-Cover Root Cause(s)

Physical

When we are working on the physical level, it's important to investigate the bodily systems, from cells to organ systems. I ordered several functional medicine specialty tests designed to get to the root cause of imbalances. We started with food sensitivity testing, adrenal and hormone testing, stool testing, and a comprehensive metabolic urine test. These test results would take a few weeks to come back, so while we were waiting for the laboratory data, I told Mica we would work with her diet.

Food can be toxic or it can be medicine. I put her on a food plan that eliminated common inflammatory foods and gave her a plan that focused on clean proteins and 9-12 cups of a variety of vegetables per day, making sure she was "eating the rainbow." I explained the connection between her hypervigilant immune system and her gut. I then showed her how the perception of overwhelming stress is what activates her fight-or-flight response system. We talked about how managing the perceptions of her stress would have a direct influence not only on her gut and genetics, but also on her hormone balance. I then began asking her questions related to the mental root cause area.

Mental

Not surprisingly, given the intense inflammatory response Mica's body was having, I discovered she had suffered several kinds of abuse in her childhood. She had been a victim of physical, emotional, and sexual abuse, as well as severe neglect. Her fight-or-flight stress response system had been activated at an early age, and she remained in a constant state of vigilance, always scanning to make sure she and her children were safe. Given her history, this was exactly what the wise mind of her child-self needed to do in order to feel safe. However, in adulthood she *was* safe and didn't realize it. She had never been asked to confront these early beliefs and therefore they were still actively controlling her adrenal and hormone system each time she went into fight-or-flight stress response. She had a rigid thought system that was causing rigidity in her body.

All of this made sense to Mica. Her misery-to-motivation ratio was such that she was willing to give anything a try at this point in her life. She was tired of the steroid roller coaster and of never knowing when her body was going to go off. She felt she lived inside of a time bomb. She agreed to do trauma release therapy.

Emotional

When I explored Mica's emotional life with her, it turned out she had a lot of drama in her family. She was easily angered and often felt betrayed by those she loved. Anger is the hard crust that covers a softer feeling. When we broke through the crust, Mica cried, letting out years of stored hurt, fear, anxiety, and panic. She could see how these emotions were triggering her stress response system and contributing to her hormone imbalance, insomnia, leaky gut, immune issues, and joint pain.

I taught her how to find the places in her body where she felt strong emotions. At first, she couldn't connect to her body. She only "felt" her feelings in her head. Gradually, she began to connect, perhaps for the first time, with where her emotions were tethered inside her body. She was challenged often in therapy to confront her beliefs, but resisted giving up the structure that she believed had kept her safe for so long. Eventually, as the rigidity of her black-and-white beliefs began to soften, so did her anger and resistance to self-inquiry.

Spiritual

Mica was raised Catholic, had attended Catholic schools, and as an adult had an intense hatred for the church, for the religious idea of God, and for anything that smacked of spirituality. Again, we uncovered anger, this time with God.

If God was so loving, how come there was so much suffering on the planet? Why did innocent children have to endure so much pain? Where was the fairness in this whole God story? Once again, Mica bravely agreed to confront her childhood meanings and beliefs in order to reverse her autoimmunity. (We'll be covering the tools Mica learned later, in Section IV. You'll get to work with those tools, too.)

Story

Mica had felt abandoned and betrayed by her mother, her father, God, and life from a very early age. Her first memories of abuse went back to pre-verbal infancy. There was plenty of evidence to support Mica's belief that the world was an unsafe, unpredictable, and terrifying place, because for her it was. Her life was threatened by her mother and her father during separate instances of child abuse. She was neglected, told she would never amount to anything, and taken out of high school before she finished. She grew up in abject poverty and was ashamed of everything about her life. It took several therapy sessions for her to connect to her little girl self in a compassionate way. She was so filled with self-loathing that when she got connected to her little child self, she only wanted to kill her. This level of self-hatred comes from severe abuse. It is not possible for you to recover from this without a good trauma release therapist.

All therapy styles are not the same, and all therapists are not equally qualified or good at their jobs. Talk therapy is not helpful for re-wiring the brain after trauma. Trauma release techniques, such as clinical hypnotherapy, Eye Movement Desensitization Reprograming (EMDR), and Brainspotting are all proven techniques for post-traumatic stress disorder (PTSD) and for helping the brain turn down its sensitivity for fight-or-flight activation after severe stress. You could call trauma from abuse capital "T" trauma, and sustained perceived daily life stress lower case "t" trauma. Both have the same impact on the brain. The brain is damaged after "T" AND "t" traumas. This is why I tell anyone who has been diagnosed with autoimmune disease to begin trauma release therapy.

Take a look at the following checklist and see if any of these apply to you. If you check even one, you are a candidate for one of the styles of therapy I mentioned above.

- Your feelings and emotions are too intense for you or those around you to manage.
- You are ruminating about a hurt or trauma and can't stop.
- You're using a food, shopping, gambling, or an addictive substance to cope.
- You can't focus or concentrate at work or at home.
- You feel disconnected from activities or people you used to love.
- Your relationships are strained or filled with drama.
- Your friends have told you they're concerned about your behavior.
- You cannot stop a self-defeating behavior or thought pattern in spite of trying your hardest.
- You are picking fights or bullying those around you.
- You are blaming circumstances, people, or the world for your current situation.
- You feel powerless in some area of your life.
- You feel listless, bored, and unable to take care of the basic activities of daily living that need to be handled.
- You are not eating.
- You are not sleeping.
- You cannot manage your emotions.
- You have compulsive and obsessive thought patterns.
- You have gone through a loss such as a romantic break up, a move, a job transition, a death, or the loss of a pet or loved one other than due to death.
- You have received an autoimmune diagnosis, a diagnosis of cancer, or any other health-related crisis for you or someone you love.
- You have recently had an upsetting or high-stress event in your life.
- You need emergency help if you are cutting yourself, thinking of harming others or yourself, or have a plan for harming others or for suicide.[2]

---

[2] Need help? In the U.S., call 1-800-273-8255 for the National Suicide Prevention Lifeline.

Mica's story indicated she needed trauma release therapy. If I had focused on her hormone complaints and not noticed the welts on her skin, who knows where Mica would be today. She did get the therapy she needed. Today, when a big crisis arises in her life, Mica still stresses and struggles not to lash out at God. She questions what she has learned about energy. She questions the miraculous visions she has had in her meditations and the connection she has formed with her higher Self. This is the frightened child part of herself. But she now has tools for reaching that powerless part of herself and she no longer wants to kill her inner child. Instead, she can self-soothe in a way she was unable to do three years ago.

Step Two: Confront the Data

Just to recap, we un-**C**overed the root causes of Mica's autoimmune disease in all 5 root cause areas: physical, mental, emotional, spiritual and within her story. She had triggers in every one of the four corner puzzle pieces. When we ran her **genetics**, we found she had several genes that, if triggered, would set off her immune system. She had **leaky gut**. She was sensitive to many **environmental toxins** and, like everyone today, was exposed to them daily. And finally, she had **trauma** in her childhood.

Mica was able to **C**onfront the data we collected, feeling relieved that there was something that could be done to reverse her autoimmune disease. Many of my patients are not upset to find that, like Mica, they have food sensitivities, intestinal bugs, adrenal and hormone imbalances, and nutritional deficiencies in addition to their leaky gut. When they receive SAM model bloodwork back and are told that "nothing is wrong," they despair. Mica had lived through this experience many times. She was elated to see lab result data that reflected how she was feeling.

Step Three: Connect the Dots

One month after her initial visit, Mica's hives were gone, she was sleeping through the night, her mood was lighter, and she had lost some weight. She was cautiously hopeful. It was time to **C**onnect the dots. This is when you begin to see how your thought patterns, eating habits, and lifestyle choices inform your level of vitality and wellness. After a week on a clean diet, Mica was seeing the connections. She saw that garbage in will mean garbage out. Food=Mood. She was reversing her autoimmune disease.

Over the next year, she killed off gut infections, got well on her way to healing her leaky gut, balanced her hormones and adrenal glands and began metabolizing her thoughts and nutrients more efficiently. She was on several nutritional supplements that were speeding her recovery. She remained in therapy and began slowly chipping away at the layers of self-loathing we were uncovering from her early abuse.

Step Four: Create the Life You Desire

As she began to heal energetically, mentally, emotionally and physically she realized how much of her life she was living in a reactive state rather than a proactive state. She saw that her childhood beliefs had created unhealthy default strategies that she had used to cope with her stress. She had eaten a lot of sugar, watched a lot of television, and worried about everyone in her life except herself. Now, slowly, she was creating strategies that were intentional and meaningful for the stage of life she was in.

She learned the importance of self-care and began loving and connecting to herself. I call this upgrading your operating system from the factory default settings. She was, and still is, Creating her life with intention. In this fourth step of the Freedom Framework, there is no end-point. You are never finished. It's the continuation of self-confrontation, self-inquiry, and self-realization. And now Mica is doing it without an autoimmune disease to get in her way.

For your healing, I have created a program to help you repair the damage from chronic life stress, old emotional wounds, and past childhood and adult trauma. It's called You Un-Broken. It's online and when you purchase it you will also be part of a beautiful tribe of women who are also doing this work in a private Facebook community. I hope you will join us there. It takes a village to heal that hurt child. You can register for it in the Resources Section.

CHAPTER 5

Puzzle Piece Two-Leaky Gut

"If there's no breaking then there's no healing, and if there's no healing then there's no learning."

~ONE TREE HILL

Deborah

Deborah, a 32-year-old Hispanic woman with multiple sclerosis (MS) came to see me when her medications stopped controlling her symptoms. Deborah had been diagnosed with MS 10 years prior to her first visit with me. In those 10 years, she had gone from energetically mothering her 2 daughters, running marathons with her girlfriends, and traveling on wine tasting excursions with her husband, to "dragging" herself "from point A to point B" as she told me through tears. Her last brain imaging scan had shown an increase in brain lesions, which explained why she was having new bladder, bowel, and muscle spasticity issues. As her symptoms progressed, her libido level was tanking and her depression and anxiety were rising.

Step One: Un-Cover Root Cause(s)

Physical

Deborah's disease had been developing for many years. She had been diagnosed 10 years before I met her, but she had been developing MS for far longer than that. She already had brain changes and organ damage. She was on a long list of medications, all targeting her equally long list of symptoms. She was now suffering from many of the side-effects of her medications. This is often the case. She started feeling dizzy after beginning her newest prescription medication. In response to her query, her doctor had told her to "Hang in there; it will probably pass." That was two years before she came to me, and it had not passed.

The adverse side effects to prescription medications can often be worse than the original ailment. Prescription drugs cause nearly 52% of American deaths. This number comes from actual autopsies. It is believed the real number is much higher. If you are taking four or more medications, the rate of negative complications, including death, increases exponentially.

The CDC has declared prescription drug abuse an epidemic in the United States. There are several reasons we are facing this crisis. One is the relationship between the insurance industry, the pharmaceutical industry, and the Uncle SAM model. Another is people blindly following a doctor's advice rather than listening to their own bodies. This is usually based on a fear response that understandably kicks in when your body isn't functioning the way you expect it to. The third reason is the idea that prescription medications are "free." In truth, there is a cost to taking medications that are toxic to the body. For example, hydrocodone, a prescription opiate commonly prescribed for pain, is synthetic heroin. The brain and the body see this drug in the same way they see heroin. We are creating heroin addicts when we put people on opioid medications for pain.

In looking for physical root causes, I ordered laboratory tests similar to those I had ordered for Mica, but added a comprehensive genetic work up. I put her on a mild liver detoxification protocol and an eating plan that included 12 cups of vegetables daily, 6 of which I had her juice first thing in the morning. As I do with all my patients who love their alcohol and coffee, I asked her how likely it would be that she would be able to eliminate both for a period of time while we worked on reducing her inflammatory state. Because her misery was so high, she readily agreed and indicated high motivation for doing whatever she needed to do.

Deborah told me one of the main reasons she had come to see me was because she wanted off her medications. She had heard from someone in her social circle that I had helped them get off their meds and they had never felt better. As I told Deborah, and I will now say to you dear reader, never take yourself off your medications!

Once the body has become dependent on drugs, it will react badly if you just stop taking them. You might then come up with the conclusion that your body can no longer function without these drugs. This is likely not true, but it is true that you need to be weaned slowly of all prescription medications. It is also important to work with a functional medicine provider who knows how to replace them with a nutrient or nutrients that will strengthen you rather than create a health crisis for you. When you have a broken leg, you don't just throw your crutches away. You strengthen the leg before you can walk and run again. It's a slow and deliberate process. This is the same for ridding yourself of your prescription medications. It is possible; it just must be done correctly so you succeed.

Mental

Deborah was feeling mentally "defeated." She believed her body had betrayed her. She had an expectation that if she ran daily for exercise, ate well, and took care of herself, she would never get sick. Her disease had shattered the premise she had built her life on. She felt "broken" and was grieving for her previously healthy body and her youthful vitality. She felt disgusted by her weakened bowel and bladder function and was angry when her muscles didn't behave the way she wanted them to. Deborah was a driven perfectionist who didn't believe she was a perfectionist because she judged herself as "so very far from perfect."

She had been raised by a father who wanted her to succeed in ways he himself had not succeeded. She believed her father only loved her if she was excelling at whatever she did. Failure was not an option in her world. She did not permit herself to make mistakes and she certainly couldn't abide a body that was failing in her eyes. She had never considered the idea that MS was the very teacher that life had brought her so she could release a belief that was impossible to live up to. If you believe you must be perfect to be worthy of love, will you ever succeed in consistently being loved? If your body is imperfect, will you be able to love it if perfection is the expected outcome of all you do?

Emotional

Deborah was in a state of panic that she refused to acknowledge to anyone, including herself. Her fear permeated every bit of her language. She started her sentences with, "I'm afraid that ____" (my husband will leave me, my kids won't want to hang out with me, my friends will stop calling me, I'm not going to be able to get my old life back). For the last 10 years, she had hidden these fears and never spoken of them to anyone, trying to live her life like nothing was wrong.

When I pointed out the panic implicit in her wording, she became angry, believing I didn't understand what it was like to have a body with a bankrupt health account. With tears welling up in my own eyes as I felt her pain, I told her my story of having had rheumatoid arthritis. I also let her know that the very anger and fear she had been expressing in my office was contributing to the advancement of her disease. She responded, "So you're saying this is my fault?"

This response from Deborah is not unusual. People don't like to be blamed for anything that goes wrong. It can bring up shame. Deborah was feeling shamed by me in that moment because she was projecting blame and judgement from me that was not there. In reality, Deborah had been blaming herself. She had been berating her body for not allowing her to live up to her standards of what it meant to be a "good wife, a good mother, a good friend."

As I explained to Deborah, giving up the idea that someone or something has to be at fault is the liberating shift needed to stop rigid thinking. No one was to blame for Deborah's development of MS. Not her childhood, not her genetics, not her exposure to toxins, not her lifestyle habits, not the medications she was on; there was no single element that had caused her autoimmunity. The critical mass of many factors had caused her boat to capsize. There were several pieces to her puzzle that caused her body to tip from balance into imbalance. Symptoms are just feedback from your body; that's all. They are feedback that something you are doing is not working for you. If you listen carefully to your body, it will inform you when you need to make a change. If you medicate it, ignore it, or judge it, your symptoms will just get louder as the imbalance moves deeper into your tissues.

The unfortunate part of Deborah's story is that no one taught her this in the early days of her diagnosis. She was taking the information her body was giving her and creating a story about it. She wanted her "old life back." This is never possible. We cannot return to the past. We can, however, create an even better future, which is just what Deborah did.

Spiritual

As I continued my interview with Deborah, I discovered she was a devout Christian who attended church at least once a week, and often more. Deborah believed that if she had enough faith, God would heal her. She judged herself as faithless because her disease was progressing. Eventually, Deborah got clear that she was seeing God as she did her biological father: someone who was never going to love her until she did everything "right." Again, she had set herself an impossible task to accomplish.

I am not saying that God doesn't heal and there are no miracles. I have witnessed miracles countless times. I am saying she had not considered that her symptoms were feedback. She was not considering the idea that MS was a series of symptoms that had developed because the root causes had not been addressed. She was not considering that she herself had the responsibility to listen to her body, pay attention to her body's language, and to love her body. How could she, though, if her childhood belief that she had to be perfect to deserve love was driving her? She wanted God to listen to her, but she wouldn't listen to herself.

I asked her if she believed that God helped she who helped herself. I asked if she believed that God wanted her to be a participant in the solution to her puzzle. She acknowledged that theoretically she believed this, but realized she had not been living that way. She wanted God to just make her suffering go away. I knew we were getting somewhere at that point.

Story

Deborah's belief that she had to prove herself perfect to be worthy of love, both on planet earth and in Heaven, was formed in early childhood before her brain was fully developed. She had felt criticized by her father and could recall several incidents of being humiliated in front of others as a result of his criticism. This is a form of trauma. Throughout Deborah's childhood, her father smoked heavily, both in the house and car. Deborah's mother had rheumatoid arthritis and her father had psoriasis. All four of the corner pieces of Deborah's puzzle were in place—genetics, leaky gut, toxins, and trauma—as was the frame. It was time to work on the middle using the 5 R's.

Step Two: Confront the Data

Deborah's genetic results revealed she had a difficult time with metabolizing estrogen and with part of her detoxification pathways. She had multiple issues with her immune function and in some of her energy production systems. This means the multiple environmental pollutants, which act as estrogen mimickers, were creating more toxicity than she could handle or get rid of. Her cellular energy production was already handicapped, and with the extra load her detoxification organ had, it was no wonder her disease was progressing. We ran some additional tests and found several areas that would respond well to incremental lifestyle changes and nutritional supplementation.

One of the areas that Deborah changed as a result of her testing was her alcohol consumption. She looked at her genetics, her laboratory data, and could see how damaging her passion for wine was to her health. She once again became angry in my office, feeling victimized because this was "the one thing" she and her husband did together for fun still. "What else will you make me give up so I can't have fun?" she asked me plaintively. I explained again, this was feedback from her own body. It's not anyone telling her what she can and cannot do. This way of thinking is not uncommon in women with autoimmune disease. The need to judge, blame, and shift responsibility outward in order to remain powerless and victimized keeps you from being able to end your autoimmune disease. It is what is called a secondary gain for holding onto your disease.

Secondary gains are the benefits of remaining chronically ill. Most people don't consciously believe they benefit from being sick. However, in chronic illness, there is usually a subconscious need to remain ill. For example, in women with chronic migraines, I will ask if they voluntarily take time out to rest or do they only go to bed in a dark room when a migraine makes it mandatory. I often hear a wry response that acknowledges some truth to this statement. No, they don't voluntarily take time out for themselves. They have to be sick before they do that. Sometimes a woman will remember the only attention she got from her mother in childhood was when she was sick. Now, in adulthood, she will get the attention of her spouse, friends, or community if she is sick.

It is essential to look for secondary gains to your autoimmune disease. They are there. If you do not find and address them, you will not be able to reverse your disease.

Step Three: Connect the Dots

Deborah discovered the connection between her secondary gain needs, her love for wine, diet, her beliefs, her frequently internalized anger, and her current state of health. She responded quickly to the quick-start program I put her on, as it reduced the toxic burden on her body. Her depression, anxiety, and internalized anger began to lift as she did the work I gave her for releasing trauma and changing her belief patterns. As she connected to her inner child self in a more loving and patient way, her relationship with God shifted. She began to feel loved and accepted by God and found that going to church became a time of real communion rather than a time of begging to be released from what she saw as punishment in the form of autoimmune disease.

We weaned her off her medications, one at a time. She worked with a pelvic floor specialist and learned biofeedback methods for tuning into her body. The more she took on the responsibility for listening to her body, and connected the dots between her thoughts, food, and actions, the more attuned she became. The more attuned she became to her body, mind, heart and spirit, the more her symptoms abated. The more relief she got from her symptoms, the more she trusted her body, God, and life.

One year after beginning her program, she had another MRI. She had no new lesions and had regained the full use of her bowels, bladder, and muscles.

Deborah had reversed her autoimmunity by understanding the corner pieces of her puzzle, framing her puzzle, and then working with the center of the puzzle using the 5 R's: 1) **R**emove, 2) **R**eplace, 3) **R**epair, 4) **R**e-inoculate, and 5) **R**ebalance.

1. **Remove:** She had removed toxic thoughts, toxic skin care products, toxic medications, and toxic foods from her life.

2. **Replace:** She had replaced wine with fruit infused water, coffee with capomo, impossible beliefs with nurturing beliefs, toxic medications and foods with an abundance of nutritious vegetables, and clean protein and supplements targeted to reverse her imbalances.

3. **Repair:** Deborah repaired her relationship with her family of origin, using her adult brain and forming new beliefs. She had been unable to do this with the old thought pattern of judgement, blame, and criticism. More importantly to her, she repaired her relationship with God. She finally felt that the mental theory she had heard in church all of her life, that God loved her, was actually true. She could feel it from her spirit to her cells. It felt like a giant "cosmic hug" each time she connected to God. She hugged me every time she remembered how unworthy she had previously felt of God's love.

4. **Re-inoculate:** The new belief that Deborah re-inoculated herself with was, "I am enough just as I am. I am perfect in my imperfections. I know that I only learn through my mistakes and I encourage myself to get out there and get messy. All of it IS God."

5. **Rebalance:** Deborah had to examine her life in terms of energy expenditure the same way she looked at her financial spending and saving. She knew she had overdrawn her body's health account. She was deeply in debt when she came to see me. The program I put her on allowed her to tuck some energy away in her health account. But when she went on vacation 6 months into her program, she came home with muscle weakness and pain again. She had overspent her energy. She was frightened when she saw me, afraid she wouldn't regain the progress she had made.

I explained that the body reallocates resources to maintain balance. That means it will rob Peter to pay Paul until Peter has nothing left to give. When that happens, you will get symptoms of an energy deficit. Just like having an overdrawn bank account, you will have to spend time on a strict budget to build your health account back up. When you have a nice cushion, you don't have to be as strict, but you still need to be careful to keep your accounts balanced.

Deborah stopped saying yes to everything she was asked to do. She started advocating for herself. She also began to implement a daily routine that included self-care, self-connection, and self-communication.

Step Four: Create the Life You Desire

Deborah, like me and so many other women who are on the other side of autoimmune disease or cancer, is now grateful for her disease. She knows her MS served as a catalyst to really change the beliefs and lifestyle choices that were not working for her. She found the restorative yoga I prescribed for her was so helpful, she went through yoga teacher training and now volunteers as a yoga teacher for women who have MS.

When I asked her a year into her recovery if she would like to have her "old life" back, she laughed and told me that she was now living a life she could not have even imagined the year before. Her "new life" included freedom from the mind traps she had set for herself in her childhood. She was empowered and helping other women to become empowered. She was fulfilled in a way she had not been even before her MS diagnosis. MS had truly been not only a wake-up call, but a gift.

What Is Leaky Gut?

The term leaky gut syndrome is also known as intestinal permeability syndrome. Just for clarification, leaky gut is not leaky butt. I often have patients who tell me they do not have leaky gut because their rectal sphincter is working just fine. When your intestinal lining becomes porous, undigested food molecules, yeast, toxins, and other waste products that would not normally get through what is supposed to be a contained system, escape freely into your bloodstream.

Remember, your intestinal lining is the first line of defense for your immune system. The exterior layers of intestinal cells, or epithelial cells, are linked by "tight junctions." The microvilli at the ends of these cells aid in the absorption of digested nutrients and then send them into the bloodstream. If these tight junctions loosen, the gut lining will become porous and allow molecules to flow directly into the bloodstream.

Once these molecules escape into the bloodstream, your immune system mounts an attack. Your liver will try to screen out the "foreign invaders" that the damaged intestinal wall can no longer hold back. The waste, undigested food, and microbial toxins that enter the bloodstream as a result of leaky gut wind up in the liver, whose job it is to detoxify and dump these poisons. Under ordinary circumstances, the liver is taxed just by processing the daily waste created by cell and organ activity. With leaky gut, there is a larger load. Eventually the liver becomes saturated and is incapable of this level of detoxification, so toxins are returned to the bloodstream.

The blood will filter as much of the extra toxicity as it can. The lymphatic system will then attempt to collect and neutralize the toxins, but unable to send the toxins to the liver, the body eventually becomes toxic. Microbes then reproduce and create chronic lymphatic swelling, especially in children. Eventually, toxins will collect in the tissue around muscles and joints, causing joint and muscle pain which can eventually settle in as fibromyalgia. If the toxins settle into the cells, this inflammatory process can lead to genetic mutations and ultimately cancer.

The immune system is now in over-drive, fighting off perceived antigens and creating antibodies left and right. Picture the old Space Invaders video game from the 1980s. Now you get the picture. As the immune system sustains its attack, inflammation is the byproduct of the war going on. Your body is fighting itself by fighting what you eat. Your joints might begin to hurt, your skin could develop a rash, you will likely feel fatigued and gain extra weight. If this process goes unchecked, you will begin to develop auto-immune disease as each layer of tissue becomes more and more inflamed. You will be more sensitive to chemicals, foods (even those you used to be able to eat), the environment, and susceptible to infections such as the Epstein-Barr virus. You could develop sinus congestion, itchy ears, digestive issues, brain fog, and headaches.

If you take a look at *figure 16*, you will see this process illustrated.

▼ **Figure 16**

Leaky gut and the progress to autoimmune disease and cancer

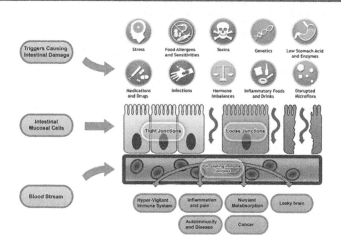

What Causes Leaky Gut?

Your gut wall houses 70 percent of the cells that make up your immune system. This is why 5,000 years ago, it was written in Ayurvedic texts that the root of all disease (and wellness) starts in the digestive system. These early healers knew that digestive problems are linked to autoimmunity, aller-gies, fatigue, weight problems, mood disorders like depression and anxiety, sleep difficulties, dementia, and cancer. The gastrointestinal system affects the entire body and is now called our second genome. Yes, it even impacts how we express our genetics.

You have over 100 trillion microscopic organisms living in your gut that can be organized into 500 different species. These little critters account for 3–5 pounds of your body weight and help you break down your food and keep your gut wall healthy. Even in a perfect world, your gut has a hard time keeping you balanced and your digestion running smoothly. In the frenetic and fast-paced world we live in today, filled with fast food, eating on the run, and over-booked schedules, a number of factors can tip the balance towards leaky gut.

Here are some of the most common causes of leaky gut:

- **Medications:** Acid-blocking drugs, chemotherapy, steroids, anti-inflammatories, antibiotics, and the oral birth control pill can damage the gut wall and inhibit healthy digestion.

- **The Standard American (SAD) diet:** Our calorie-rich, nutrient-poor diet of processed foods causes the wrong bacteria and yeast to grow in the gut, leading to an unhealthy gut ecosystem.

- **Toxins:** Mercury fillings, chemicals in the environment, home, personal hygiene products, and your mattress, and mold toxins can create a toxic overload that can damage the gut lining.

- **Low stomach acid and digestive enzymes:** Stress, the removal of your gall bladder, a deficiency in zinc and other minerals, and acid-blocking medications can all impair proper enzyme and stomach acid production.

- **Gut infections:** Yeast, small intestinal bacteria overgrowth (SIBO), parasites, and a bacteria called heliobacter pylori can all impact your digestive function, and consequently your immune function.

- **Stress:** The stress hormone cortisol released by the adrenal glands when you are under chronic stress will alter your gut nervous system and break down your gut lining. This is a primary cause of leaky gut and an unhealthy ecosystem of gut microbes.

- **Food sensitivities and inflammatory foods:** With leaky gut, nutrients are absorbed before they are fully digested. The body's immune system will tag some of these foods as foreign invaders. The body sees the inflammatory reaction of your immune system to these foods as yet another stressful event, causing more gut-wall-destroying cortisol to be released from your adrenal glands. And so the cycle continues.

- **Infections:** When the gut lining is damaged, the body is more vulnerable to bacterial, fungal, parasitic, and viral infections, which become resistant to treatment. These resistant microbes cause doctors to prescribe more and more antibiotics, which causes candida (yeast) overgrowth. Candida causes more gut-wall inflammation, and so the vicious cycle continues. With the gut wall now more and more permeable, or leaky, the yeast and bacteria can escape into the bloodstream and settle into any area of the body, including the brain, sinuses, bladder, vaginal wall, and skin.

- **Hormonal imbalances:** Leaky gut can cause a problem with blood-sugar regulation, which can cause a decrease in testosterone and an increase in estrogen in men, putting them at risk for muscle wasting, weight gain, and prostate cancer. The same issue can cause an increase in testosterone and an increase in the wrong kind of estrogen in women. This increase in testosterone in women can lead to hair loss from the head, extra hair on the face, weight issues, and infertility. The increase in estrogen can put women at risk for estrogen-related cancers.

Most of us are subject to one or more of these factors, which is why leaky gut is so common. In fact, every one of my clients has leaky gut to some extent. That means undigested food molecules escape into the bloodstream and activate the immune system, which is wired to attack anything it senses that is "not you." This attack leads to inflammation, which can show up in a host of ways, eventually developing into any number of diseases. It's a hypervigilant immune system that creates "auto-immunity" or "you attacking you." You are indeed what you eat, and if your immune system is not friends with what you eat, it turns on you in a variety of ways (*see figure 17*).

How to Fix Leaky Gut

The most common symptom I see in my patients with autoimmune disease, and therefore leaky gut, is multiple food sensitivities. When partially digested food proteins work their way through your gut wall and into your bloodstream, your immune system will rightly take offense. Your immune system is wired to attack anything that is "not you." This offensive reaction will mean you develop food sensitivities that will multiply in number and severity the longer you do not treat your leaky gut.

▼ Figure 17

How leaky gut affects the entire body

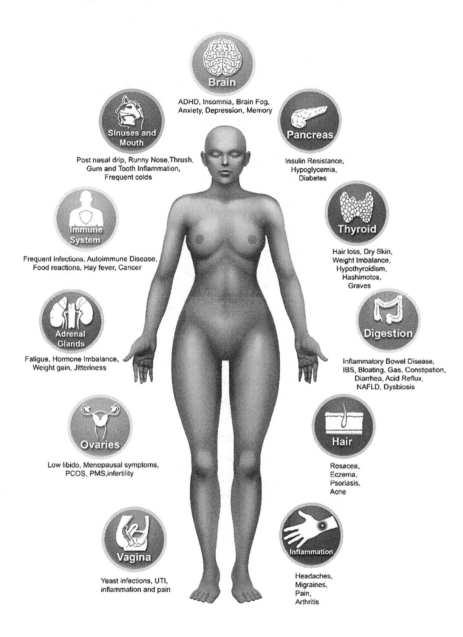

Food Allergies vs. Food Sensitivities

Food sensitivities are not necessarily food allergies. When your lips go numb or you break out in hives anywhere from 20 minutes to two hours after eating a food, this is known as an IgE (immunoglobulin E) *food allergy*. This can be picked up when you go to see your allergist, who will run a radioallergosorbent blood test (RAST) and/or a skin allergy test. These tests do not detect IgG (immunoglobulin G) reactions from your immune system.

A food sensitivity is a non-IgE reaction, which is characterized by the measurement of IgG antibodies to food proteins not tolerated in a person's body. An IgG food sensitivity is a delayed hypersensitivity reaction. It can take four hours to four days for symptoms, silent or overt, to appear after eating the offending food. This distinction is often lost on the Uncle SAM model of healthcare. IgG food sensitivity testing is often dismissed as invalid because, like IgE testing, it is limited.

IgG testing only measures one mechanism of the immune response. There are often several non-immune responses, such as a histamine intolerance and gut wall damage from lectins, in people with autoimmune disease. I use Mediator Release Testing (MRT) to make sure as many factors are tested for that could be creating critical mass for the body. The release of mediators like histamines, cytokines, or prostaglandins from the white blood cells are usually triggered by the activation of the immune system, whether it's IgG, IgE, IgA, IgM or a complement reaction.

The complexity of the immune system makes food sensitivity testing controversial. I have found the MRT methodology simplifies the leaky gut healing process and covers the most bases.

As listed above, there are many causes for leaky gut, but they can be distilled down to four main categories: 1) food, 2) stress, 3) toxins, and 4) bacterial imbalances/infections. Let's start with food.

The SAD Food Program

Sugar, GMO's, pasteurized dairy, gluten, and the phytates and lectins found in grains and soy are the most common foods that cause inflammation and damage your intestinal lining. Sprouting and fermenting grains reduces phytates and lectins, which can make some of these grains more digestible. However, when you are embarking on a program to heal leaky gut, it's best to just stay away from these foods.

Unfortunately, many households have gotten used to the standard American diet (SAD) program that includes eating from cans, packages, boxes, and fast-food restaurants, which pack their products with leaky-gut causing ingredients. Better to go from SAD to GLAD (Gluten-free, Lectin-free, All-natural Diet). There are several versions of GLAD programs popular right now. Some are vegan or vegetarian. Others are paleo, autoimmune paleo, or more specific, such as the Specific Carbohydrate Diet. Others use a dosha-specific Ayurvedic plan. I have found that, like everything else in life, there is no one size that fits everyone.

Choosing the Right Food Plan for You

No matter where you are on the autoimmune spectrum, there are certain foods in the SAD that are not good for anyone, and I recommend you eliminate them completely. If you choose to indulge very occasionally in a favorite item on this list, please do it slowly and mindfully with love and joy and avoid consuming it fearfully.

One of the most damaging eating disorders functional medicine has propagated is called orthorexia. Orthorexia is anxious and obsessive behavior in pursuit of a healthy diet. This eating disorder creates so much fear that people who suffer from it begin to think of food as an enemy. Specific foods are classified as good or bad. What orthorexics don't realize is that, like anorexia or bulimia, this obsessive and adversarial relationship with food causes the *4F stress response system* to engage right at meal time. Meal time is when you want your 4F life-support system online so you can digest and absorb and eliminate properly.

The items I am going to recommend you eliminate from your diet are not to be classified as "bad"; just think of them as non-foods. When I talk about whole foods, nourishing foods, disease-reversing foods, I am talking about the food your great grandparents likely ate if they had a garden and lived close to the land. Much of what we call food today is not even food. The definition of food is, *any nutritious substance that people eat or drink in order to maintain life and growth*. The substances I am asking you to remove from your diet are not food, and therefore are not contributing to life or growth for you, but rather disease and deterioration.

FOOD = MOOD

FRUIT+VEGGIES+PROTEIN ⟶ HAPPY

SUGAR+PROCESSED FOOD +ALCOHOL+CAFFEINE ⟶ DEPRESSION, ANXIETY AND FATIGUE

Non-Foods to Eliminate to Flourish and Thrive

- Gluten
- Processed, packaged, boxed, canned items
- Pasteurized, non-organic dairy products
- Sugar, high fructose corn syrup, and other artificial sweeteners
- Chemicals such as added flavoring, artificial coloring, preservatives
- Toxins from contaminated farmed animals and fish
- Products that come from animals that have been treated with cruelty
- Hydrogenated and trans fats
- Alcohol
- GMOs and non-organic foods
- Stimulants such as caffeine
- Depressants such as marijuana

Further Foods to Eliminate if You Have Leaky Gut

- Grains (you can add sprouted versions of non-gluten containing grains later in the healing process)
- Legumes (you can add sprouted versions in later in the healing process)

- Natural sweeteners from coconut, maple, rice, dates, agave, stevia, and xylitol (in the beginning of your healing)
- Soy
- High glycemic index fruit (*see Table 2*)
- Vegetables high in starch (*see Table 2*)
- Meats that have been treated with antibiotics and chemicals and raised inhumanely
- Eggs
- Tomatoes, white potatoes, & eggplants
- Peppers including bell peppers and hot peppers
- Spices such as curries, paprika, and chili powder
- Nuts and seeds
- Fried or fast food
- Chocolate
- Dried fruit

What to Eat

- 10-12 cups of vegetables that encompass the whole rainbow of color
- Bone broth
- Clean protein with every meal
- One serving of low glycemic fruit per day
- Raw organic honey for infrequent sweetening
- Organic herbal tea and infusions
- Healthy fats such as ghee, coconut oil, and avocados
- Plenty of herb infused, fruit infused, or plain water
- Fresh herbs and spices other than the ones I listed above

The glycemic index ranks foods on a scale of 0 to 100 based on how fast it causes an increase in blood sugar. Foods that with a high number raise blood sugar quickly, and foods with a low number are slower to impact blood sugar levels.

The GI is divided into three categories, so you can pay attention on keeping your blood sugar even rather than having to obsess about numbers. The three categories are:

GI of 55 or less = low
GI of 56 to 69 = medium
GI of 70 or more = high

The goal is to balance any high-GI foods with foods lower in GI in order to remain satiated and energized while maintaining a stable blood sugar. The Glycemic Index Charts that follow are for you to get a visual for how much sugar is in the food you are eating. If you are trying to lose weight, kill off gut pathogens, or balance your blood sugar, this is a wonderful tool for you to use. There are foods listed on these charts that are processed, contain gluten, and are grains. I included them to give you an idea of how much sugar they contain.

The lists I just gave you are by no means exhaustive. This is to give you an introduction to the impact food has on your gut. For a more detailed and deeper dive, I have written the Whole Individualized Life Detox (WILD) Program that takes you through five modules that include more information than can fit into one book. In the WILD Program, I give you more detailed information on healing emotional wounds, leaky gut, detoxification and diet. For example, you will get downloadable lists for healthy food swaps, healthy fats and oils, a shopping list so you can begin to clean out your pantry and stock it with nutrient dense foods, and tips, tricks and recipes for replacing your favorite non-food items. You can also sign up for the free 21-Day Quick Start Program and begin your journey to autoimmune reversal immediately. Information about both the WILD Program and the free bonus material is in the resources section of this book.

Will you be cured in 21 days? No. I don't talk about curing your autoimmunity, but rather reversing it. Why? Because if you follow the program I give you and begin to feel better, reverse your inflammatory and autoimmune markers, but then revert to your old ways of emotional reactivity, self-limiting beliefs and behaviors and non-nourishing dietary choices, you will find yourself living with fatigue, weight problems, mood issues, inflammatory symptoms, and autoimmune disease again.

Remember the misery-to-motivation ratio? This is never so pronounced as when we talk about diet. I always test for food sensitivities in my patients with autoimmunity, and I repeat the test every 9–12 months while we are actively healing their leaky gut with supplements, food programs, emotional healing, and mental reframing.

I will often hear my new patients tell me they have already tried getting rid of gluten, and it "didn't work." You must have realistic expectations when you are healing a problem that may have been in place for decades. If you eliminate only gluten for a couple of weeks and don't feel better, it's because

▼ Table 2: Glycemic Index ratings of a variety of foods

FRUITS

Food	GI Value
Cherries	22
Grapefruit	25
Prunes	29
Apricots, dried	30
Apple	38
Peach, canned in juice	38
Pear, fresh	38
Plum	39
Strawberries	40
Orange, Navel	42
Peach, fresh	42
Pear, canned	43
Grapes	46
Mango	51
Banana	52
Fruit Cocktail	55
Papaya	56
Raisins	56
Apricots, fresh	57
Kiwi	58
Figs, dried	61
Apricots, canned	64
Cantaloupe	65
Pineapple, fresh	66
Watermelon	72
Dates	103

VEGETABLES

Food	GI Value
Broccoli	10
Cabbage	10
Lettuce	10
Mushrooms	10
Onions	10
Red Peppers	10
Carrots	49
Green peas	48
Corn, fresh	60
Beets	64
Pumpkin	75
Parsnips	97

BEANS

Food	GI Value
Chana Dal	8
Chickpeas, dried	28
Kidney Beans, dried	28
Lentils	29
Lima Beans (frozen)	32
Yellow Split Peas	32
Chickpeas, canned	42
Blackeyed Peas, canned	42
Baked Beans	48
Kidney Beans, canned	52

SWEETENERS

Food	GI Value
Stevia	0
Yacon syrup	1
xylitol	12
Fructose	19
Coconut palm sugar	35
Brown rice syrup	45
Marmalade	48
Honey	55
Evaporated cane juice	55
Molasses	55
Sorghum syrup	55
High fructose corn syrup	58
Jam	65
Brown sugar	65
Sucrose (white sugar)	68
Maple Syrup	76

CRACKERS

Food	GI Value
Stoned Wheat Thins	67
Ryvita Crispbread	69
Melba Toast	70
Kavli Crispbread	71
Soda Crackers	74
Graham Crackers	74
Water crackers	78
Rice Cakes	82
Rice Crackers	91

SNACKS

Food	GI Value
Hummus	6
Peanuts	15
Walnuts	15
Cashews	22
M & M Peanut Candies	33
Milk Chocolate	43
Potato Chips	57
Kudos Bar	62
Corn Chips	63
Popcorn	72
Jelly Beans	78
Pretzels	83

POTATOES

Food	GI Value
Yam	37
Sweet	44
New	57
Canned	65
White skinned mashed	70
French Fries	75
Baked	85
Instant Mashed	86
Red Skinned, boiled	88

CEREALS

Food	GI Value
Muesli	43
Bran Buds	47
Oat Bran	55
Bran Chex	58
Raisin Bran	61
Cream of Wheat	66
Quick (One Minute) Oats	66
Pancakes	67
Puffed Wheat	67
Special K	69
Grapenuts	71
Bran Flakes	74
Cheerios	74
Cream of Wheat Instant	74
Shredded Wheat	75
Waffles	76
Rice Krispies	82
Corn Chex	83
Corn Flakes	92

PASTA

Food	GI Value
Fettuccini (egg)	32
Spaghetti, whole wheat	37
Spaghetti, white	38
Star Pastina	38
Spiral Pasta	43
Capellini	45
Linguine	46
Macaroni	47
Rice vermicelli	58

GRAINS

Food	GI Value
Barley, pearled	25
Converted, White	38
Long grain, White	44
Buckwheat	54
Brown	55
Basmati	58
Couscous	65
Cornmeal	68
Aborio	69
Short grain, White	72
Instant, White	87
Wild rice	87
Glutinous (Sticky)	98

BREADS

Food	GI Value
Pumpernickel	41
Sourdough	53
Stone Ground whole wheat	53
Pita, whole wheat	57
Whole Meal Rye	58
Hamburger bun	61
Croissant	67
Taco Shell	68
White	70
Bagel	72
Kaiser roll	73
Bread stuffing	74
Whole wheat (100%)	77
French Baguette	95

two weeks isn't long enough and gluten isn't the only thing you needed to eliminate. I start with the lists I gave you in Table 2 and then begin to fine tune to the individual. For example, genetic testing indicates what diet your individual body wants you to follow: vegetarian or paleo style.

If you are miserable with severe digestive symptoms and cannot tolerate many foods already, then start on a Specific Carbohydrate Diet™ (SCD) plan. If your misery level is mild, start with a paleo diet, utilizing the food list I provided above. If your genetics indicate meat puts you at a higher risk for heart disease and Alzheimer's disease, then modify both the SCD and the paleo diet to include wild fish as your source of meat protein, collagen, and egg white protein. Yes, collagen and egg whites come from animals. Collagen is also processed. However, neither contains the animal fats that a person with an APOe 4/4 gene cannot metabolize well (more on this in the WILD Program).

The Specific Carbohydrate Diet

The Specific Carbohydrate Diet (SCD) was developed in the 1950s by Dr. Sidney Haas. Yes, as far back as the 1950s people were struggling with celiac and other autoimmune diseases. Dr. Haas treated the young daughter of Elaine Gottschall, who then went on to write the book that helped me reverse the worst of my oldest son's Asperger's Syndrome 45 years later. The name of the book is *Breaking the Vicious Cycle.*

The SCD is a program that removes processed, GMO, sugary and starchy products from your diet. It has been used by thousands of people in the last 70+ years to heal digestive, immune, and mental imbalances. Like Ayurvedic medicine, the SCD principles consider that we are not all the same. Not every digestive tract can digest man-made chemicals and highly processed carbohydrates and sugars. Any improperly digested carbohydrate can be used as food for unwelcome gut microbes, such as yeast, bacteria, or parasites. When an overgrowth of any of these organisms occurs, they reproduce by using the sugars you feed them and then release toxins and acids into your digestive system, which can cause damage and inhibit nutrient absorption and the proper elimination of waste. The build-up of these acids and toxins then creates the vicious cycle that worsens leaky gut.

The SCD eliminates these sugars, thus cutting the organisms off from their food supply, and then begins to restore gut flora so the intestinal wall can begin to heal as inflammation is reduced.

The SCD is introduced using easy-to-digest foods and progresses with more complex foods as the gut heals. It can be individualized to fit your specific digestive state of injury or health. The idea is that as your inflammation reduces, gut walls repair, healthy flora balance is restored, and disease is reversed, your food options will expand as your tolerance expands.

Stress, Toxins, and Bacteria

The other three primary causes of leaky gut—stress, toxins and bacteria—will be covered in later chapters. Toxins and bacterial infections are the subject of the next chapter, where you are going to meet another amazing patient of mine, Penny.

Healing leaky gut takes patience and time. Later in the book I will give you some tips to get your started. However, it really can take years as you go through the layers of healing infections, detoxing from toxic exposure, and repairing the microflora balance in your intestines. I created the **WILD (Whole Individualized Life Detox) Program** for this purpose. It includes the **You Un-Broken** course when you purchase the WILD program because I want to make sure you are detoxing properly from your emotional pollutants too. You can register for the WILD Program in the Resources Section of this book. When you do, you will join a whole tribe of WILD Women who are all supporting one another in their journey to slimmer, sexier, and supercharged in 30 days!

CHAPTER 6

Puzzle Piece Three– Environmental Toxicity

"There is no life to be found in violence. Every act of violence brings us closer to death. Whether it's the mundane violence we do to our bodies by overeating toxic food or drink or the extreme violence of child abuse, domestic warfare, life-threatening poverty, addiction, or state terrorism."

~BELL HOOKS

The third corner piece of the autoimmune puzzle is exposure to environmental toxins and *toxicants*. A toxicant is a man-made substance that has been introduced to the environment. Examples of toxicants are pesticides, industrial pollutants, bisphenol and the millions of other toxic chemicals being introduced into our environment every year. A *toxin* is poisonous substance produced in nature that can cause disease when introduced into the body. Examples of toxins are infections such as the Epstein-Barr virus, yeast or bacterial overgrowth in the intestinal tract, and exposure to allergens and molds.

One often over-looked source of toxicity is from us humans. We can be in toxic relationships, have toxic habits, expose ourselves to toxic media, and be in toxic work environments with people that are toxic.

Health and vitality is a result of a simple formula: Your individual genetics, plus your exposure to toxins, plus your ability to detox those toxins (including the mental and emotional ones), plus your digestive health will result in your unique level of health.

LEVEL OF VITALITY = GENETICS+ TOXIC EXPOSURE+ ABILITY TO DETOX+ DIGESTIVE HEALTH

Before we go into more depth regarding these various forms of ubiquitous toxins, I would like to introduce you to Penny. Notice the many types of toxic exposure in Penny's life as I take you through solving her autoimmune puzzle by using the Freedom Framework process.

Penny

Penny was 28 years old when she came to see me with chronic fatigue, hypothyroidism, constipation, and joint pain. She was on several prescription medications and had been to multiple doctors, none of whom had diagnosed her with autoimmune disease. Penny said, "she was at the end of her rope." She had no libido and her fiancé was getting frustrated with their lack of sex life and that they were no longer able to do the physically demanding activities that had first brought them together.

Step One: Un-Cover Root Cause(s)

Physical

Penny had been diagnosed with hypothyroidism in high school shortly after her parents were divorced. She had been on a synthetic form of T4 ever since. Her "regular doctor" only monitored her TSH (thyroid stimulating hormone). Her joint pain began while she was in college, 6 months after getting date raped. She had been constipated "forever" (since childhood). She made the decision to come and see me because a friend at work had told her that I had helped balance her hormones and energy and had encouraged her to check me out. She was there because she "couldn't get out of bed in the morning." She and her fiancé smoked pot 3–4 evenings a week to relax after work. On the nights she didn't smoke, she drank 1–2 beers or glasses of wine. She didn't eat sugar (not realizing that's what beer and wine are) and worked out 5–6 days a week, but it "wiped her out."

I ordered the same laboratory tests I had ordered for Mica and Deborah, which included the comprehensive thyroid work up, autoimmune/inflammatory markers, and bacterial and viral screen I do for everyone I see. I also put her on the same eating plan. Are you seeing a pattern? Remember autoimmune diseases, regardless of the name, are all in the same bucket with the same choices of root causes. When I am working to solve the autoimmune puzzle for a patient, I am looking at the four corner pieces and putting together the frame. I also asked her to stop working out so hard for the time being, encouraging her to instead go for daily walks in the woods near where she lived.

Mental

My inquiry then turned to the time well before her parents' divorce. Divorce doesn't happen suddenly. There is usually discord in the home between parents before they finally make the decision to split up. I asked her to recall the first time she could remember not feeling like her parental unit was unified. She brought up a memory of them fighting when she was three years old. I asked her what meaning she had applied to that event. She told me she didn't feel like she could get air when she breathed, like her belly was in knots and she wouldn't survive. I asked her if her constipation started there and she burst into tears.

Constipation is literally holding onto your sh*t. As children, we are unable to express feelings of panic in a way adults can understand. Penny had learned to hold it all in. She also believed she could fix her parent's marriage if she was "good enough." She became a classic people pleaser. She also began a pattern of co-dependence in her relationships and was living that out with her current fiancé as a result of that childhood meaning, belief, and behavior.

Emotional

Penny cried easily. She did not hold her emotions back; she held her truth back. She was unable to express what she thought authentically for fear that she would be abandoned by those she loved. She created relationships with men that demanded more of her than they gave back. She was attracting men that would leave her if she set boundaries. What she had not confronted and therefore not realized was that she trained them to be this way. By not setting good boundaries, she notified her boyfriends, and now her fiancé, that she was there to take care of their every need. This is true for many women with thyroid disease, especially early onset thyroid disease. Again, there is often trauma and a distorted childhood belief that makes it nearly impossible for them to speak up authentically.

I pointed out the relationship between Penny's beliefs and perceptions and her brain and relay system, of which the thyroid is a part. When the fight-or-flight response is activated because someone pushed her button that set off self-defeating childhood beliefs, the adrenal glands release the stress hormone cortisol. This in turn can decrease the conversion of T4 to T3 and reduce TSH, thus creating thyroid hormone resistance. In addition, over time the cortisol will break down the gut lining and her joint tissue.

Spiritual

Penny was Native American, but had no connection to her tribal culture. We spoke at length about how grounding this relationship would be for her. Again, she cried as she recounted the multiple moves her family had made after her father had lost his job when she was young. She felt she had no roots and had not thought about reaching out to her family's tribe. She was filled with hope at the thought of connecting to her ancestral spirituality and heritage.

Story

Penny filled out the Health Map as homework and found the exercise was helpful in giving her a bird's-eye view of her whole life and the contributing factors that had gotten her to where she was that day. Her story included toxins (alcohol), trauma (divorce and rape), all of which were impacting her genetic expression and the development of leaky gut and subsequent autoimmune disease.

Step Two: Confront the Data

Penny's laboratory data revealed she had autoimmune thyroid disease or Hashimoto's thyroiditis. Like many women I see, she had a second auto-immune disease, mixed connective tissue disease (MCT). In addition, she had a yeast overgrowth in her intestines, was positive for an active Epstein-Barr virus infection, and had a severe adrenal and hormone imbalance. It is worthwhile to mention here that I have never seen anyone with leaky gut not have Epstein-Barr virus (EBV). Penny had mononucleosis in her adolescence, which had left her with EBV. The CDC reports that 90% of Americans carry EBV. It's implicated in chronic fatigue syndrome and flares when there is acute stress.

Step Three: Connect the Dots

Penny discovered the connection between her diet, her past trauma, her beliefs, and her current state of health. She discovered that the research linking marijuana and alcohol use to waking up in the middle of the night was relevant to her insomnia. She could easily fall asleep after the use of pot and alcohol, but could not stay asleep. Over the next year, she would struggle with her addiction, quitting until her joint pain lifted, and then resuming the next time she had a stressful period in her life, causing her joint pain to return.

Eventually, she agreed to start psychotherapy for trauma release. The second year after her diagnosis, she got sober and has stayed sober ever since. She found her addiction to coffee to be the toughest to recover from. Seeing her thyroid autoantibodies go down to zero and her MCT reverse, she went back to her coffee habit. Remember the misery-to-motivation ratio? That's the problem with getting better; we often feel it's then okay to go back to the habits that caused our problems. Fortunately, in Penny's case, when she saw her autoantibodies elevate again, she realized the connection between what she put in her mouth and how her immune system behaved. She quit coffee again.

Step Four: Create the Life You Desire

As Penny worked on her codependency with food, she also worked with her codependent relationships with her job, her family of origin, and her fiancé. She is now married. Her fiancé, now husband, was willing to do couples counseling with Penny and they are the proud parents of a baby daughter who is healthy and happy. Penny's puzzle included all four of the cornerstone triggers: genetics, leaky gut, toxins, and trauma. By framing her puzzle using the Freedom Framework, she methodically, one step at a time, reversed her autoimmunity. Is it gone forever? No. She can reactivate it if she takes her attention from the pieces of her puzzle we had discovered together.

Food as a Source of Toxicity

When you have leaky gut, food is a source of toxicity and autoimmune triggering. Food proteins that make their way through the gut wall and into the bloodstream will cause an inflammatory response in the body as the immune system reacts to what it sees as a foreign invader. This might be gluten, dairy, soy, or sugar, but it could also be broccoli, blueberries, salmon, or coconut oil. This is why the MRT food sensitivity testing discussed in Chapter 5 is so important. However, if you have already stopped eating gluten, dairy, soy, alcohol, and sugar and they don't come up reactive on your food sensitivity testing, this does not mean you should be eating them.

When you have leaky gut, what you are eating a lot of will typically show up on your test results—especially if you are not rotating your foods. Why have I not seen any signs or symptoms of RA in myself for over 20 years? Because I don't eat gluten, dairy, soy, sugar, alcohol, or processed foods. I don't eat grains. I don't eat candy. I don't drink soda, ever. I eat whole foods that are nutrient dense. I can do little to control the air I breathe or the pollutants that occur outside of my home. But I *can* control what I put in my mouth. Know this: there is nothing you are eating or drinking that does not fall into one of two categories: inflammatory or not inflammatory. Because I know there is no grey area, I know the food on my fork or the beverage in my cup will either promote life or it will poison me. It is up to you to choose.

People as a Source of Toxicity

People can also be toxic. You might have a toxic work or home environment filled with drama. Toxic relationships drain vitality and activate the 4F stress response system. You might even have some toxic behavior patterns or habits of your own. In Chapter 4, I covered the autoimmune connection to past toxic experiences or trauma. Just as chemicals, allergens, and infections create changes in your physiology and genetic expression, so does trauma and emotional toxicity.

Therefore, not only are you *allowed* to terminate toxic relationships, but to reverse your inflammation and autoimmunity, you must. If you need permission to walk away from someone who is hurting you, I am giving it to you right now. Do it. If you don't, you will continue to kill yourself slowly. Get angry, be selfish, and allow yourself to be unforgiving for now. You don't owe anyone an explanation for taking care of yourself. We will work on the next step later, the forgiving of yourself and those who have hurt you.

I consider much of what is in the media quite toxic. I have learned to limit my exposure to certain kinds of movies and avoid television completely. I have had patients come into my office in a state of panic over political elections, a football game, or a headline in the news. I always gently point out that the activation of the 4F stress response system as a reaction to events or people that you have no control over will cause a worsening of inflammation and autoimmunity in the body. A rigid mind will lead to a rigid body, which ends in injury and pain. Limiting your exposure to all toxicants, including toxic situations and media helps to keep critical mass low so your body doesn't capsize. We will talk later about how to detox from the harmful effects of built up toxicity. A media fast is a wonderful thing to do during your detoxification program.

Infections as a Source of Toxicity

Bacterial and viral infections impact the autoimmune response by a process called molecular mimicry. Molecular mimicry is a structural, functional, or immunological similarity between infectious pathogens and your own body. The infectious agent can then blend into the host. Parasitic infections can create inflammation in this way, which can then lead to an autoimmune response.

Research is ongoing as scientists search for connections between infections and autoimmune disease. No single organism has been found to be responsible for the development of autoimmune disease. Scientists have found that several different infections can be present in a single autoimmune disorder. Some examples of infections and the related autoimmune diseases are:

- **Rheumatoid arthritis:** Epstein-Barr virus (EBV), hepatitis C virus, Escherichia coli bacteria, mycobacteria
- **Lupus:** EBV
- **Multiple sclerosis:** EBV and measles virus
- **Myasthenia gravis:** hepatitis C virus, herpes simplex virus
- **Guillain-Barré syndrome:** EBV, cytomegalovirus (CMV), Campylobacter bacteria
- **Type 1 diabetes:** Coxsackievirus B4, mumps virus, CMV, and rubella virus
- **Myocarditis:** CB3, CMV, chlamydia

Please note, not everyone who has had these infections will develop auto-immunity. As you have learned, it is usually a build-up of risk factors from all four cornerstone pieces of the autoimmune puzzle, including a genetic predisposition, that leads to autoimmune disease.

Chemical Toxicants

The endocrine system is a network of glands that produce hormones that tell the body what to do. Chemicals that interrupt this process are called endocrine disruptors. Typically, estrogen-mimicking toxicants attach to the estrogen receptors present in a woman's body and interfere with the hormone dance. This interference can lead to infertility, hormone imbalances, loss of memory, learning difficulties, obesity, mood imbalances, autoimmune disease, and several kinds of cancer, such as breast cancer. These toxicants also alter how our genes are expressed, which can then be passed through to later generations. The damage due to the weak regulation of chemicals introduced into our environment is long term and often irreversible.

Women Are Velcro for Chemical Toxicants

Only 10% of the nearly 13,000 chemicals used in cosmetics have been evaluated by the US Food and Drug Administration (FDA) for safety. Even today, cosmetics are released into the marketplace without having to receive FDA approval or to share safety information. So even if the label on your shampoo, nail polish, deodorant, or moisturizer claims to be non-toxic, it likely isn't. There is no oversight. Just because it's in the marketplace, doesn't mean it's safe to use. When the FDA does finally deem a chemical such as bisphenol A (BPA) unsafe, it is removed from products by the manufacturers only to be replaced with other just as toxic chemicals. There are now many BPA-free products. However, manufacturers who have charged more money for their "healthy" BPA-free products, have just replaced BPA with BPS or bisphenol S, which is at least as toxic as BPA, if not more so.

Take a look in your bathroom and purse. If you are the average American woman, you use 12 different personal care products (including cosmetics) per day. These products contain an average of 168 different chemicals, which you are absorbing through your skin. When you apply anything to your skin, it is the same as if you ate it. Think about the last time you put an antibiotic cream on a cut, diaper rash ointment on your child's bottom, applied bug spray or stuck a hormone patch on your body. Yep, it's absorbed.

Women absorb a whopping five pounds of makeup through their skin a year, which can contain 16 different hormone-altering chemicals, such as phthalates and parabens. Makeup also contains shocking amounts of lead, arsenic, thallium, and cadmium. This chemical soup, made from plastics, pharmaceuticals, feminine hygiene products, personal care items, and the chemicals in our homes, offices, schools, cars, air, water, food, and clothing is now believed to be one of the reasons women are going into earlier menopause than the generations before. It's certainly a factor for the higher incidence of autoimmune disease in women than in men.

The Environmental Working Group (EWG)

The EWG is a non-profit, non-partisan organization dedicated to protecting human health and the environment. As such, it is a great resource for you to use to keep up on the latest research and safety data on environmental toxicants. When you visit ewg.org, you will find the following information right at your fingertips:

- The Skin Deep Guide to Cosmetics, which explains what the chemicals you see listed on your personal care and cosmetic product labels really are and what they can do to you.
- The Clean 15 and Dirty Dozen Shopper's Guides to picking produce.
- Water-filter purchasing tips.
- How to buy safe seafood.
- A Food Score app.
- A healthy cleaning guide and label decoder.
- A healthy home tip guide.
- A Safer Cell Phone use guide.
- The Dirty Dozen endocrine disruptor list.
- How to avoid buying GMOs.
- Sun screen guide.
- Children's cereal guide.
- Light bulb guide.
- Bug repellant guide.

Detoxing

"Reducing carbon emissions is important, but it is short-sighted if not coupled with reducing the toxic emissions from our heart; and that is something spiritual leaders are supposed to teach and something all thinking people, regardless of their beliefs, should practice."

~RADHANATH SWAMI

One puzzle piece at a time

It's impossible to eliminate and avoid every toxic chemical in your environment. Please note that your body is a dumping ground for the toxicants that are ubiquitous in our air, water, soil, food, household products, personal-care products, cars, garages, homes, medicine cabinets, playgrounds and work places, toys, and clothing. Little by little these toxicants build up and begin to interfere with hormone signaling and genetic expression, creating inflammation and eventually autoimmunity in your body. Consciously and intentionally limiting your exposure is a great start. Use Table 3 to guide you in swapping out the poisons in your home for safe products.

▼ **Table 3:** Safe product swaps for detoxing your environment

THE POISONOUS TOXICANT	THE SAFE SWAP
Non-stick and aluminum cookware.	Switch over to glass or ceramic.
Plastic goods: wrap, baggies, bottles, and storage containers.	Switch over to glass.
Feminine hygiene products, such as tampons and sanitary pads.	A reusable soft sided menstrual cup or reusable organic cotton pads.
Commercial shampoo, moisturizers, toothpaste, antiperspirants, sunscreens, and cosmetics usually contain parabens, phthalates, and other poisonous chemicals.	The Environmental Working Group's (EWG) Skin Deep database is a great resource for finding personal care products that are safe.

THE POISONOUS TOXICANT	THE SAFE SWAP
Vinyl shower curtain.	Glass door or cloth curtain.
Fabric softeners and dryer sheets.	Dryer balls, homemade dryer sheets with a couple of drops of essential oils, add vinegar to your wash, or wear natural fabrics that don't gather static.
Contaminated house dust is a source of toxic flame-retardant chemicals.	Vacuum frequently using a vacuum cleaner with a HEPA filter.
Furniture, carpeting, pillows, linens, and clothing that are treated with flame-retardant chemicals.	Purchase furniture, pillows, carpets, linens, and clothing that are made from leather, cotton, silk, wool, and Kevlar, which are naturally more fire resistant.
Avoid stain and water-resistant carpet, clothing, and furniture treated with perfluorinated chemicals (PFCs).	Purchase furniture, pillows, carpets, linens, and clothing made from leather, cotton, silk, wool, and Kevlar.
Plastic baby toys, books, pacifiers, teething rings and bottles.	Use glass, stainless steel, or silicone for bottles and oral products. Replace plastic dolls with cloth ones. Use bamboo and wood when appropriate.
Cleaning products that contain chemicals such as 2-butoxyethanol (EGBE) and methoxydiglycol (DEGME).	Make your own vinegar and water with essential-oil-based cleaning solutions or purchase chemical and fragrance-free products.
Insect repellants and pesticides.	Mix water and witch hazel with insect-repelling essential oils, such as citronella, lemongrass, eucalyptus, rosemary, tea-tree oil, cedar, lavender, and mint. Pour into a spray bottle and apply without fear.
Non-organic meat.	Select pastured, sustainably raised meats and dairy to avoid exposure to hormones, fertilizers, and pesticides.
Milk and dairy products treated with the genetically engineered recombinant bovine growth hormone (rBGH or rBST).	Make your own flax seed milk, hemp milk, coconut milk, sesame seed milk, or almond milk.
Farm-raised fish, which can be contaminated with PCBs and mercury.	Eat only wild-caught fish.
Bath and drinking water from the tap.	Use a whole house reverse osmosis water filter to eliminate or at least reduce toxins such as fluoride and chloride.

THE POISONOUS TOXICANT	THE SAFE SWAP
Processed, canned, and packaged foods.	Locally grown, in-season, organic, whole foods. Make sure to wash all produce well.
Medications, such as antibiotics, the birth-control pill and non-steroidal, anti-inflammatory drugs (NSAIDs).	Explore biofeedback, Ayurveda, aromatherapy, acupressure and acupuncture, homeopathy, and chiropractic medicine before reaching for drugs. Keep your immune system healthy by eating a diet full of nutrient dense vegetables, proteins, fats, and complex carbohydrates. Use turmeric as an anti-inflammatory and get fitted for a diaphragm for birth control. Meditate and exercise. Reserve antibiotics and NSAIDs for when you absolutely need them.
Recreational drugs such as marijuana.	Learn to meditate.
Alcohol	Use herbal infused waters, fizzy drinks sweetened with stevia and free of flavorings and coloring, or kombucha.
Stimulants such as caffeine.	Use Capomo (see resource section) or herbal teas.

Only when you are ready

The word detoxification, or detox for short, is over used. Due to the monumental mass of toxins and toxicants we are exposed to, we all seem to know we need to clean out periodically. But how and when? Again, there is no one-size-fits-all answer to that question. Thousands of years ago, Ayurvedic medicine began recommending detoxification with every season change. If people were guided to rinse the body's filters that long ago, when our environment and foods were relatively pure, imagine how much we need it today.

However, Ayurveda does not tell every person to detox in the same way. There are several feedback mechanisms from the body that, if listened to, can guide you through a safe detox journey. Just be sure you don't get on what I call the detox-retox rollercoaster. In other words, once you have done a cleansing program, be sure not to immediately revert back to the toxic habits and substances that polluted your system in the first place.

Here are some factors to check in with to see if you are ready for a detox:

- Do you have the time, energy, and motivation to adhere to a program that will require your focus? If the answer is yes, read on.

- Are you financially able to purchase the foods and supplements needed? Plan on $100-$250 every 3 months to do a thorough cleanse. The price depends on what is going on with your individual health. If the answer is yes, read on.

- Are you committed to yourself and your health? If the answer is yes, read on.

- Do you have severe skin, digestive, adrenal, mood, sleep issues, or are you in a great deal of pain? If the answer is yes, you need a gentle detoxification program with some supervision.

- Has testing confirmed you are carrying heavy metals in your teeth, bones, and tissues? If the answer is yes, you need to strengthen your adrenal health and kill off gut pathogens before you start a medically supervised chelation program with a trained professional.

- Have you been detoxing regularly already and this is not your first rodeo? If the answer is yes, you might want to do some testing to see where your organ systems are. Pancha Karma, the Ayurvedic detox of queens, might be a great option for you.

Any detox program must include detoxification of your mind and heart while you are cleansing your body systems. When done regularly, this will help keep you connected to spirit and the collective unconscious, where all wisdom is contained.

This book cannot guide you through a supervised detoxification program. As I mentioned in the last chapter, I have created a program that allows you to individualize your detox and get some supervision in an online group setting. It's called the Whole Individual Life Detox, or WILD Program. The WILD program takes you through a step-by-step process in much greater detail and depth than what I can provide here. If you are not ready to commit to yourself on that scale, you can sign up for my 21-Day Quick Start Program (see resources section). I will send you 21 emails that will encourage you to start laying the foundation for a deeper dive later. These 21 days will get you going with self-care habits that I teach to every single patient who sees me in my clinic.

Now let's move to the final corner piece of the autoimmune puzzle, genetics. You will meet lovely little Tiffani, a young girl who had her autoimmune disease reversed thanks to a diligent and motivated mother.

CHAPTER 7

Puzzle Piece Four-Genetics

"Your genetics load the gun. Your lifestyle pulls the trigger."

~MEHMET OZ

Your body is composed of between 10 and 50 trillion cells. Your intestinal tract contains over 100 trillion bacteria. This means the 3–5 pounds of microscopic critters that live in your gut outnumber the cells that make your body up by as much as 10:1. They have a huge influence on how your genetics are expressed. But I'm getting ahead of myself. First, let's do a little simple science and review what this whole genetic thing is all about. Why are genetics important when we are trying to solve the puzzle of inflammation and autoimmune disease?

A Brief Synopsis of Genes and How They Function

To begin with, each of your trillions of cells has a central command station, or nucleus. Each nucleus contains 46 molecules called chromosomes. You get 23 of those from your mother and 23 from your father. These contain the instructions for how to build you. If you zoom in on your chromosomes with an electron microscope, you will find that each is made of bundles of tightly coiled loops. Unravel the coils and a six-foot long double strand of deoxyribonucleic acid, or what is known in shorthand as DNA, is revealed.

A gene is a bit of DNA. You have approximately 23,000 genes. DNA is often pictured as a ladder. Each rung of the ladder is a pair of nucleotides. There are four types of DNA nucleotides that are reported on lab tests using the letters A, C, G, and T, which are short for adenine, cytosine, guanine, and thymine. You have an impressive six billion pairs of these nucleotides in each one of your cells. Your genes are the blueprint for how your body runs itself. Genes do all of this by making proteins that then take care of the functions that keep you alive. Over 100,000 different proteins are responsible for digestion, the immune system, circulation, cell signaling and communication, movement and much more.

These all-important proteins are created by enzymes, which transcribe your DNA code and then build a strand of nucleotides called mRNA or messenger RNA.

This complex genetic sequence can be simplified by just remembering that DNA is used to make RNA. Then RNA is used to created proteins, and proteins, which are made from amino acids, do all of the heavy lifting in the body. Interestingly, researchers now know that less than 2% of your DNA actually codes for proteins. The remaining 98% is all about regulating the expression of your genes. This is where the science of epigenetics steps in.

Epigenetics is the study of changes in organisms caused by modification of gene *expression* rather than alteration of the genetic code itself. In other words, that 98% of genetic material that science used to call junk, is a powerful factor in determining your state of health, level of vitality, and how well your immune system works.

DNA is perpetually subject to mutations, or changes to its code. These mutations can cause malformed or even absent proteins, which can lead to disease. A mutation is called a single nucleotide polymorphism, or SNP for short. We all start out our lives with SNPs that are inherited from our parents and are known as germ-line mutations. You can also acquire SNPs during your lifetime, which you can then pass on to your offspring. Some of these mutations occur during cell division and others are caused by damage from toxicants such as chemicals or trauma, or toxins like bacteria or viruses that opportunistically take up residence when you have leaky gut.

And now we have come full circle with all four of the corner pieces of the autoimmune puzzle. Your genetics, just like your exposure to environmental toxins, traumatic life events, and leaky gut, do not act by themselves. These four factors are intimately connected, and if autoimmune disease is to be reversed, they must all four be addressed.

I want to introduce you to a young patient of mine named Tiffani. Tiffani's autoimmune disease was largely influenced by her mother's micro-biome, which became her first microbial gut population during her trip through the birth canal when she entered the world. Her genetics were then influenced by this microbial soup that did not start out as a healthy ecosystem because her mother's wasn't healthy when she was born.

Tiffani

Tiffani is a 5-year-old African American girl, the second of three daughters in her family, who was brought to see me by her mother. Tiffani's mother had recently given birth to her third daughter. Shortly before the birth of the new baby, Tiffani began breaking out in a rash on her legs, arms, back, and buttocks that kept her awake at night scratching. She soon became oppositional in her behavior and defiant with her mother. Tiffani's mother had taken her to several doctors who had all diagnosed the rash as eczema and prescribed steroid creams, which worked temporarily at best. Tiffani and her mother were beset with stress, both losing sleep, and feeling drained and exhausted.

Step One: Un-Cover Root Cause(s)

Physical

We tested Tiffani for food sensitivities. Mom had already tried to eliminate gluten, dairy, and sugar, but Tiffani was becoming more and more obstinate and was refusing to eat anything at all. Tiffani's mother wisely decided not to make food a power struggle in Tiffani's life. She knew the birth of the new baby was likely a stress for Tiffani and was playing a part in the physical symptoms she was struggling with.

I then asked Tiffani's mother if there was any autoimmune disease in the family. Yes, mom had Raynaud's and Restless Leg Syndrome, which means Tiffani's mother had leaky gut when Tiffani was conceived and born. Our gut flora is populated during birth, and it comes from mom's microbes. When you have leaky gut, you do not have the healthiest microbiome. This means Tiffani was born with a microbiome that was less than optimal. Not only that, but Tiffani's mother knew she had heavy metal exposure through the mercury amalgams in her teeth. The four corner pieces of the puzzle—Tiffani's genetics, her gut flora, the trauma of having a new sister, and receiving toxins through mom's breast milk—had all triggered her own autoimmune disease. This indicates how important it is for women in our day and age to heal our own guts and detox ourselves as much as possible before conceiving and bearing children.

Mental

When a child feels displaced in the pecking order of the family, she may react in several ways. At the age of five, Tiffani was unable to express her distress, or unable to even know what was causing her distress. She just knew she was angry. She wanted the attention she'd always had from her mother, which this new interloper was stealing from her. She was acting out in a way that made sense to her, with a brain that was not yet developed enough for higher-ordered reasoning and problem solving. Tiffani's mother was aware of the dilemma, but didn't know how to help.

I had Tiffani's mother set aside time each day just for the two of them. I also suggested she take each of her older daughters out every week for one-on-one "dates." This way, each child would know they remained an important part of the family. They could still feel loved and appreciated by their mother, and know that even though life brings changes, those changes can be weathered if everyone comes together as a family unit.

Emotional

Children can be remarkably resilient emotionally. That's the good news. I taught Tiffani ways of expressing her stress (art and play therapy), tools for reducing the 4F response system in her body (resourcing and the butterfly hug), and words she could use to express her feelings when she wanted to act out. Mom started taking Tiffani out on dates. She also set boundaries with Tiffani's behavior that included a point system for positive behavior, which culminated in rewards that Tiffani chose for herself and mom had agreed on.

Spiritual

Ultimately, Tiffani felt abandoned by her parents because of the birth of the new baby. We are wired to seek safety in a community or tribe. In the early days of humanity, we knew that being alone, outside the protection of the community, was dangerous. There were many predators that could and would eat a human wandering about lost and alone. When we feel rejected, our 4F response system gets triggered and we feel that our survival is threatened—for a very good reason, it's biology. When Tiffani's fears of abandonment were dealt with in a healthy way, which included boundaries with her oppositional and defiant behaviors, she began to relax back into the family structure, believing herself once again safe, seen, and accepted. And so her eczema relaxed as well. The rash disappeared as her mind softened its panic and her nervous system calmed down.

Story

Tiffani's story wasn't very long and she had not learned how to tell it from a victim perspective. I saw her when her baby sister was just weeks old. Her mother was insightful in seeing what was going on with Tiffani and equally wise in knowing she could not allow the reactive behavior and skin to continue or they would solidify into habits. The earlier you listen, the faster you make the changes your body is begging you for, the quicker you can reverse your disease. Conversely, when you begin to identify with autoimmunity as "your ____" (fill in the blank with the disease or issue), then you have begun to own it and it will take longer to reverse. Tiffani's mom saw her daughter's angry reactions and her skin condition as feedback, didn't panic, and sought help after doing some research of her own. This quick action meant Tiffani was sleeping much better within two weeks and her eczema had disappeared completely within three months.

Step Two: Confront the Data

Tiffani had multiple food sensitivities. Her mother also had several food allergies. When I showed the color-coded bars that indicated Tiffani's immune system's reactivity to dairy, gluten, sugar, several fruits, and a handful of nuts, Tiffani was interested. I showed her that her itching was caused by the foods represented in the colors. She agreed to remove those foods from her diet for one month. I had mom work with our functional medicine nutritionist and our laser therapist. I have found that a nutritionist is invaluable for creating meal plans that mothers and children will actually follow. It does no good to hand someone who doesn't cook, has multiple food sensitivities, or feels overwhelmed a series of recipes that they don't feel capable of following.

I have health coaches I have trained in my integrative medicine health coach program who do individual consultations and teach group classes at our clinic. It is always helpful to learn how to master the food plan that will reverse your autoimmune disease in a group with other people walking the same path. They might have questions you had never thought to ask. The group also supports one another in making what are often difficult lifestyle changes. Nobody understands what you are going through better than others going through the same thing. Most of the health coaches in the Academy for Integrative Medicine have reversed their own autoimmune disease, have discovered what it feels like to live a life full of energy and free of self-limiting beliefs, and are now passionately helping others to become empowered to do the same.

Step Three: Connect the Dots

Tiffani and her mother connected the dots between the events happening at home and her eczema. Because Tiffani was only five years old, we had only a short time to make a tangible difference in her quality of life. You have a small window of time with children in terms of attention span and willingness to change. If they see that removing gluten and dairy makes a difference, you are likely going to get them to buy into a program that eliminates those foods for life. If you remove gluten for two weeks, four weeks, 3 months, and nothing substantive changes, you are at risk of losing your child's interest and willingness to collaborate in their own health. Remember, it's usually not just about gluten, and that's why removing gluten won't always make you feel 100% better. Gluten is essential to remove from your diet if you have autoimmune disease, but you have to look at the rest of the puzzle.

The pressure is high at school to conform. They are in the lunchroom with other kids who are eating a standard American diet (SAD). They play sports together and are fed junk food and toxic electrolyte drinks in plastic bottles filled with artificial chemicals as "snacks." They pass vending machines in the school hallways, participate in gluten and sugar-filled bake sales, have birthdays and holidays celebrated in the classrooms with sugary toxic junk, and are asked to sell toxic sweets as fund raisers for a variety of school and scouting activities. Your child does not want to be "different." Different means you are outside of the tribe where a saber-toothed tiger can eat you. "Different" means there is a high risk of rejection.

When my youngest daughter was in middle school, we discovered she was intolerant to dairy, sugar, and gluten. She struggled with feeling like a "weirdo" at a time of life when being weird is social suicide. I told her she had a choice. She could take on this idea that she needed to belong and eat whatever her friends ate and get sicker and sicker, or she could be a leader. I taught her to cook the foods she loved in a healthy way that removed flour, dairy, and sugar. She flourished in the kitchen. I taught her to bring her own food to her activities. By the time she was in high school, her friends' mothers were asking her to teach them to make the food she was bringing over as her sleep-over snacks. Then her friends started eating like she did, because her face glowed and her body was so healthy. She had a choice of being a victim or being a leader. She chose leader and never looked back.

With kids, I always say "test don't guess." You don't want them to lose interest and willingness to collaborate in their own health. It's vital to help them connect the dots in a clear and meaningful way they cannot help but see. The food sensitivity testing we did with Tiffani accomplished just that.

Step Four: Create the Life You Desire

Parenting includes the responsibility to provide our children tools that will help them live the life they desire. This doesn't mean giving them everything they ask for. It doesn't mean sacrificing everything to "make them happy."

Remember the quote I started the book with?

"Somebody once told me the definition of hell: On your last day on earth, the person you became will meet the person you could have become."
~ANONYMOUS

The opposite of happiness is failing to become the person you are capable of. I see parents struggle with helping their children set boundaries with foods that are toxic for them. I see parents using "treats" that are filled with chemicals, sugar, and gluten to reward them for "good behavior." Children listen. If you say something is harmful for them and then give it to them later because you are tired of listening to them beg for it, they will know you are not serious in your boundary setting. Worse yet, if you say to stay away from toxic substances commonly called food, and then eat it yourself, they won't believe you and won't trust you. You have to walk your talk. That is what Tiffani's mom did. This was a great gift to bestow on her daughter at such a tender age. Tiffani now knows she can trust her mother to keep her word; she knows certain foods just don't work in her body, and she knows that food can be medicine. What an amazing lesson to be learned for one so young.

A Brief Tour of Your Amazing Body

I have left this tour until now because I wanted to help you see the entirety of the autoimmune puzzle. I wanted you to understand how your body, mind, heart, and spirit are each equally important in solving the puzzle. Too often people come away from a book or prescribed protocol for autoimmune disease and believe it's only about food or prescription drugs. Hopefully by now you can see the complexity of your body, and at the same time, the simplicity of the Freedom Framework we are using to organize your puzzle pieces. Every part of the Whole Individualized Life Detox (WILD) Program I am going to introduce you to will integrate beautifully into your unique puzzle, allowing you to solve it effortlessly. So now, before we dive further into your genetics, let's take a few minutes and take a tour of your gorgeous body and review how it all works together. Remember, your genetic material is the blueprint for how you are put together. Now let's take a quick look at the actual construction.

The Foundation

The foundation is the load-bearing part of any structure. It's the table on which you are putting together your puzzle. A great way to get to know your foundation is through the lens of Ayurvedic medicine. This book is not about Ayurveda. However, Ayurvedic medicine provides an elegant and easy-to-use framework for understanding your body and its feedback. For this reason, I use Ayurveda in my practice. The foundation of you is illustrated in the pancha koshas.

The Pancha Koshas

Ayurveda conceptualizes human beings as consisting of 5 layers, or sheaths. In other words, you are more than just your physical body. These layers are called the pancha koshas, or five sheaths (*see figure 18*).

A simplified version of the five layers is:
- The physical body, or the one we feed, water, and take for walks.
- The energy body, also referred to as chi in Chinese medicine, prana in yoga practice, and the electromagnetic energy field in Western science.
- The emotional and mental body, or the layer of you that perceives, feels, and remembers.
- The wisdom or knowledge body, or the layer of you that discriminates, holds to values, has integrity, and intuits.
- The bliss body, or your access portal to God, the Divine Spark within and without, universal consciousness.

You will see the pancha koshas depicted in two ways. One is with the physical layer as the core or first layer. Alternatively, you will also see diagrams with the bliss body as the core.

▼ **Figure 18:** The Pancha Koshas

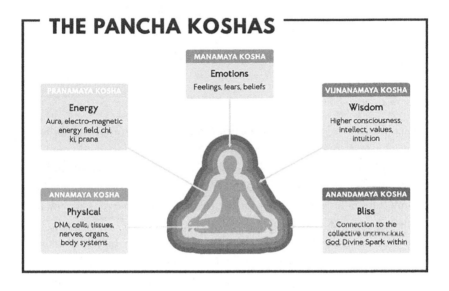

Ayurveda is wonderfully useful for helping you pick up early warning signs you are going out of balance on any level of your being. Again, in Ayurveda, digestion is considered as the source of both wellness and illness. It is the foundation of all health, and in large part of the foundation for how you express your genetics. This is echoed in traditional Chinese medicine, homeopathy, naturopathy, and even the origins of Western medicine.

Yet Ayurveda's consideration of digestion is not limited to food alone. We digest not only food, but thoughts, emotions, and spiritual and sexual experiences. What's more, each of us processes, digests, and integrates these uniquely. We react to the seasons, exercise, sexual patterns, and sleep in ways that are unique to our constitutional type or what is called our *dosha*. In Chapter 9, I will help you figure out what your body is actually trying to tell you. Check out the resources section to determine your dosha type.

The Frame

When you eat food, your digestive system breaks it down and uses the nutrients to build your tissues. According to Ayurveda, you have seven different tissue layers, or dhatus. (Do not confuse these with the koshas. These seven layers all pertain primarily to the physical body.) They are:

- Plasma
- Blood
- Muscles
- Fat
- Bones
- Nervous system
- Reproductive tissue

Each of these is built according to the health of the prior layer. In other words, if you do not get the proper nutrient-dense foods, or you do not digest and metabolize and absorb nutrients efficiently, you will not build healthy plasma. If you do not build healthy plasma, your blood will not be healthy. This in turn will affect your muscles, fat, bones, nervous system, and finally your reproductive tissue.

Further, when the digestive process is damaged, toxicity builds up in the body. Your digestive system can no longer keep up with the toxic build-up of waste through the elimination channels of the bowel, kidneys, lymph, lungs, skin, and tears. Not eliminating well is the same as not taking out your kitchen garbage. Things start to stink. This can attract vermin, like yeast, parasites, and bacterial overgrowth.

Muscles, fat, and bones are the third, fourth, and fifth layers of your structure and make up the musculoskeletal system. Your musculoskeletal system is like the frame of your house. The protein you eat is broken down into peptides and the amino acids used to build your bones and muscles. If you are not digesting properly, this is not done efficiently. Your bones store minerals and fats used by the body when it needs to access fats or minerals in times of need. They also store toxins like heavy metals to keep them from damaging your nervous system. Unfortunately, as you age and your digestive health suffers, these toxins and metals are released into the bloodstream and can damage the organ systems and nervous system. New blood and immune cells are manufactured by your bones using the stored fatty acids and minerals. This is why bone health is essential for immune health and proper metabolism.

The Electrical System

The nervous system is the sixth tissue layer of your structure. It requires healthy plasma, blood, muscles, fat, and bones to be at its best. Your body's electrical system, or nervous system, consists of the network of nerve cells and fibers that transmits nerve impulses between the parts of the body. These cells require proper fats and a perfect electrolyte solution to conduct their messages.

Your body is made from cells swimming in salt water—basically the same ratio of salt to water as the ocean. Your brain is mostly fat and the peptides gleaned from protein and runs primarily on specialized sugars. Contrary to what we thought in the 1970's, fat is not bad for you. However, fried food, trans fats, hydrogenated oils, and an unhealthy ratio of fats will not create the essential fats required for the creation and maintenance of healthy cell membranes, hormones, and the nervous system.

Fats absorb toxins, which then get into the cells. When this happens, the body needs a replacement of good healthy fats, especially if you are going to absorb the fat-soluble vitamins A, E, and D3. The proper maintenance of the fatty cell membrane is essential for the exchange of electrolytes necessary to fire the electrical impulses that power your muscles, such as your heart and even your circadian rhythm. You are an electrical being, which is why daily "grounding" is so essential. More on that in Chapter 11 when you learn how to create a grounding resource place for yourself.

The Communication System

Your circulatory and hormonal systems are both ways your body receives and generates communication. Your heart is command central of the circulatory system and your brain command central for your endocrine system. The nervous system cells, or neurons, communicate by sending nerve impulses along what are called axons. At the end of the axons, neurotransmitters are released to communicate messages to tell the rest of the body what to do. The hormones of the endocrine system also communicate complex messages, like when to have a period, when to ovulate, how to utilize the sugars you take in, and much more. Hormones are produced by endocrine glands, sent into the fluids of the tissues, and then transported to target cells mostly via the bloodstream, or circulatory system.

Endocrine System

The reproductive system is the seventh and last tissue layer in the Ayurvedic framework of your structure. The endocrine system consists of a series of glands that secrete messenger hormones, which utilize the cardiovascular system for distribution to the rest of the body. Examples of glands that are part of the endocrine system are the pituitary, hypothalamus, and pineal glands located in the brain, the thyroid and parathyroid glands located in the neck, the adrenal glands located on top of the kidneys, the pancreas located behind the stomach, the ovaries (and testes in males) located in your lower abdomen and pelvis, and the thymus located between your lungs behind your breast bone. The thymus gland plays an important role in the immune system. The hormones of the endocrine system are manufactured from fat and cholesterol.

Circulatory System

You have 10,000 miles of capillaries, or tiny veins and arteries, used to deliver nutrients and oxygenated blood and to pick up waste products to and from even the furthest reaches of your body, such as your fingers, toes, teeth and gums. When your circulatory system is sluggish, your ability to absorb the necessary nutrients required for life, from your cells to your largest organs, is inhibited. When your circulatory system is not operating efficiently, you are also unable to distribute waste to the proper elimination channels.

One of the vital elimination channels is your lymphatic system. You have more lymphatic fluid than you have blood. Your lymphatic system is responsible for cleaning up debris outside of your cells and taking it to your kidneys, lungs, intestines, and skin so they can dump the trash. Just as your heart needs exercise to keep it strong and healthy, your lymphatic system requires movement to keep it circulating and communicating with the cells. A clogged lymph system leads to a build-up of infection and toxins. In Chapter 6, I will give you tips for keeping your circulatory and lymphatic systems moving.

The Protection System

The immune system could be called your guard dog. You don't want a dog that bites everyone when they come to visit. You want your alarm system to activate only when you are truly threatened. Your immune system consists of a series of cells called T-cells, B-cells, lymphocytes and immuno-globulins that are programed to kill off invading pathogens.

Eighty percent of your immune activity occurs in your gut. You are as much as 90% bacteria, most of which is in your digestive system. This means the health of your gut microbes and your immune system are closely linked. Your immune system is balanced when your gut microbes are balanced. Dysbiosis, or imbalanced gut microbes, leads to a breakdown of your protection, or immune system. Some alarm signals that your immune system is not working properly are food sensitivities, seasonal allergies, persistent inflammation and pain, chronic sinus congestion and frequent lingering colds. Not only does your gut microbiome impact your immune system, but also your genetic expression.

This brief tour through your amazing body illustrates how the blueprint, or DNA, influences, but doesn't have rigid control over the actual construction of your structure. I use genetics in my practice to look at the blueprint, but ultimately, other functional medicine tests give me information about the state of your cellular health, digestive function, your microbiome, the efficiency of your lymph system, your levels of toxic load, and how well you are absorbing nutrients and eliminating waste. I will list these tests in Chapter 10.

The Importance of Genetics

Remember in Chapter 4 I told you that ACEs (adverse childhood experiences) can alter the structural development of your nervous system and your brain? This leads to a disruption in your messenger chemicals, or hormones, which then compromises your immune system. Early ACEs also impact your genetic expression. This is called the science of epigenetics. These epigenetic alterations happen during fetal development in utero when mom is exposed to toxins, violence, feels depressed, or even stressed.

DNA can also be altered when harmful substances enter the cells of your body and change the expression of a gene without altering the original DNA blueprint. This can result in your body repressing DNA information or expressing something that should not have been expressed, such as auto-immune disease.

The science of genetics and epigenetics is in its infancy. The information we have so far is cutting edge to us, but was recorded in ancient Ayurvedic texts thousands of years ago. What we "know" about genetics is changing daily as research brings to light more and more connections between how our genetic expression is affected by our lifestyle choices, environment, emotional health, and gut integrity. One thing we know for sure, DNA is not the only piece of the puzzle. I have found that many of my patients are afraid to know what their genetic testing will reveal. They don't want to know if they are at risk for certain diseases. In my opinion, and in my clinical practice, to know if you are at risk for certain diseases is not the reason to do genetic testing.

Why and How to Test

Knowledge is power. There are several companies that offer direct-to-consumer genetic testing. You can easily order a test online, spit in the vial and send it back. Your results will be emailed back to you within 12 weeks. The results you receive in your email may be interesting. Nevertheless, they are not useful in determining how to make lifestyle changes that will enhance your body's ability to detoxify, how to enhance methylation, or how to choose the dietary program that matches your genetic requirements.

I have my patients send their results through another portal that will extract the raw medical data that we can then use for individualizing proper diet, supplementation, and detoxification regimens. This is what individualized medicine looks like. This is not covered by insurance. No drug company will make money off this information. It's yours to use to attain your proper weight for your body type, to prevent and reverse chronic disease, to get off medications, to age with grace, to stabilize your mood, your sleep, your memory, and your energy.

It's the most exciting time in medicine I have ever witnessed. Nurtigenomics is the scientific study of the interaction of nutrition and genes, and is an important tool for true prevention or reversal of disease. It is not the only tool, but it is an efficient one.

Specific Genes Associated with Disease

We are now able to identify specific SNPs associated with liver detoxification, methylation, neurotransmitters, the immune system, your mitochondria, and much more. In my clinical practice, I use genetic testing to help my patients get off their medications for ADD/ADHD, depression, anxiety, allergies, and pain. Genetic testing is a wonderful tool I use to identify problems with weight and cholesterol management. It can even help you understand what diet is right for you and what your relationship with gluten is. However, as I have said, your genetics are only one piece of your puzzle.

There is a hard and fast rule I use when working with patients and their genetic information: *never treat the gene.* This is true for any piece of isolated laboratory data you receive. You are a unique milieu of moving parts, all trying to maintain balance in an environment ever in flux. It's important you do not take one piece of information and run with it, believing it's the smoking gun for all of your health issues.

Over the years, I have heard patients explain to me that a methylation defect is responsible for the struggles they have had throughout their years on planet earth. In the meantime, they are still eating sugar, drinking large amounts of alcohol, using marijuana to get to sleep, and blaming their parents for why they turned out the way they did. Yes, methylation plays a vital role in gene expression, liver detoxification, and brain function. It is one epigenetic factor out of many. Focusing on all of the pieces of the puzzle will allow you to solve the whole thing. Concentrating on just one piece keeps you stuck in one small, albeit very important, area.

The most important take away from this chapter is this: Your lifestyle choices impact how your genes express themselves. The gift of genetic testing allows clinicians like me to get precise in creating individualized lifestyle plans which, when combined with other elements of your story and laboratory data, give you a chance to reverse disease or at the very least halt further progression. There is no one diet that fits everyone. There is no one exercise plan, supplementation regimen, detoxification program, style of psychotherapy, or "super food" that works the same in every person. This is because we differ genetically, are exposed to different toxins, have our own unique ability to detoxify those toxins, and are digestively different from one another. Again, this is what Ayurvedic medicine taught us many thousands of years ago. Modern science is slowly catching on and catching up.

So now let's spend some time putting all these pieces of the puzzle together.

SECTION III:
Putting the Puzzle Together

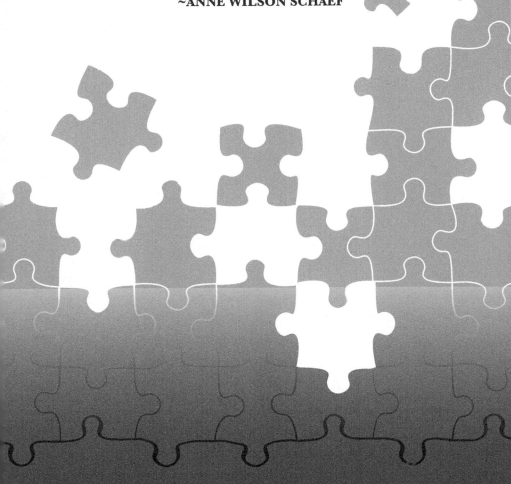

*"There are so many ways to heal.
Arrogance may have a place in technology,
but not in healing. I need to get out of
my own way if I am to heal."*

~ANNE WILSON SCHAEF

CHAPTER 8

Listening to the Feedback of Your Body

"When diet is wrong, medicine is of no use. When diet is correct, medicine is of no need."

~AYURVEDIC PROVERB

Ayurveda, a Brief Overview

To put the pieces of your puzzle together, you need to know what makes you unique. This is a gamechanger when solving your autoimmune puzzle. It explains why your friend lost weight on a food plan and you didn't. It helps you to understand that you are not broken, a train wreck, beyond salvation, or any of the other gloom-and-doom self-descriptions I hear from some of my patients who have worked with multiple doctors and tried many plans, only to remain in misery.

As I mentioned in Chapter 7, your body is an amazingly intelligent and finely designed vehicle for your spirit. Like the car that carries you around, your body also has a dashboard with feedback gauges. Perhaps you have not learned to read them yet. We are attuned to blood pressure readings, eye exams, and measuring body weight on a scale. However, there is so much more to know about your body.

I would like to take you through the feedback mechanisms your body uses to provide you with information. Information about what? About how your body is doing, when it needs more gas, whether it needs a check-up, and how much further it can go without a proper tune up—from an Ayurvedic medicine perspective.

The Three Humors or Doshas

The doshas are known as vata, pitta, and kapha. Every person is composed of a ratio of all three doshas determined at the time of conception. When the doshas are in balance, they support the normal functioning of the body; when out of balance, they create disease as they manifest in the layers of the body.

Vata

Vata is known as "king of the doshas," because when imbalanced, it can quickly imbalance the rest of the doshas. Vata is made of ether and air, and a person with a vata-predominate dosha can have the following characteristics:

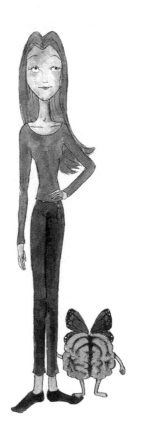

- Thin body frame
- Thin lips and hair
- Dry skin and brittle nails
- Cold hands and feet
- Creaky joints
- Learns quickly and forgets quickly
- Walks and talks fast
- Restless and scattered in mind and body
- Imaginative and creative
- Anxious and fearful
- Trouble with sleep
- Constipation
- Difficulty "staying the course" and being consistent (butterfly mind)
- Subject to mood swings

Pitta

A pitta person is the typical "type A personality" because of characteristics engendered by the predominance of fire and water elements. A person with a pitta-predominate dosha can have the following characteristics:

- Medium body frame
- Fair skin, often with freckles or moles and sensitive to the sun
- Strong appetite and digestive fire
- Warm constitution

- Early greying or baldness
- Sharp intelligence and understanding, and a curious mind
- Prone to acne, rashes, sensitive teeth, heartburn, acidity, strong body odor
- Prone to inflammation, irritability (especially in the heat or when meals are skipped), and judgement of self, which can leak out onto others

Kapha

The kapha predominate person could be called the "cookie baking mom or dad." Kapha is comprised of water and earth, which lends to the loyal stability they offer in relationships. Other characteristics can be:

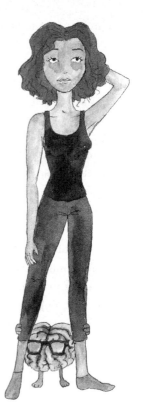

- Larger body frame with smooth, oily skin and hair
- Grounded, with slower speech and gait
- Cold skin and slow digestion
- Lubricated joints
- Learns slowly but never forgets
- Slow to get going but strong endurance
- Thick hair, nails, and skin
- Gentle and caring with a tendency toward excess weight and fat
- Copious mucus and congestion
- Prone to boils and cysts
- Sugar and salt cravings, poor carbohydrate metabolism, and frequent edema
- Sedentary lifestyle
- Attachments to love and relationships

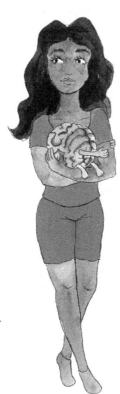

This is a very simplified overview of the 3 doshas. The best way to know your own birth mix of these doshas is to have someone skilled in Ayurvedic pulse diagnosis read your pulse. A more readily available way is to take a dosha assessment or quiz. *You can download one I use on my website at DrKeesha. com free of charge.* These assessments are not 100% accurate because many times people answer the questions according to how they feel in the moment they are taking the quiz. This only tests your dosha imbalance of the present moment. Think back to how you "usually behave" or how you would have responded at the age of 20. Another option is to have someone who knows you very well answer the questions according to what they observe in you.

Knowing your dosha balance from birth and where it is today is a great start for breaking free of imbalance and dis-ease. It becomes a guide for individualizing your interventions and lifestyle changes. There are feed-back mechanisms your body gives you to indicate your level of balance. I go deeper into reading the messages from your body in the Whole Individualized Life Detox (WILD) Program, but for now here are some quick indicators to check your own dashboard to see how your body is doing.

Your Tongue

What is your tongue trying to tell you? It is talking to you if it has any-thing besides a thin layer of saliva coating it. Your tongue should be pink, smooth, and coated with saliva only. Ancient Ayurvedic scholars called *rishis* outlined many ways to read the body. The tongue's map is seen in *figure 19.*

▼ **Figure 19:** Ayurvedic map of the tongue

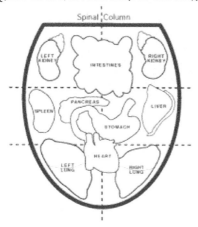

Notice where the various organs of the body are represented on the tongue's surface. If you have a coating in any of these areas, it is a sign of congestion or toxicity (called ama) in or around that organ. If your tongue is scalloped around the edges it could mean you arc not absorbing your nutrients well. If it quivers at the end when you stick it all the way out your thyroid could be imbalanced. A dry, cracked tongue can mean you have a vata imbalance. A bright, red tip can indicate a heart problem.

Checking your tongue twice a day, as you scrape it with a tongue scraper and brush your teeth, gives you feedback for further exploration. Your mouth is the first part of your digestive system. What your tongue looks like is indicative of the health of your entire digestive tract. Keeping tabs on your digestion is the same as keeping tabs on your health. Check out *figure 20* to see what your tongue is trying to tell you about your digestive health.

▼ **Figure 20:** Examples of imbalances as shown on the tongue

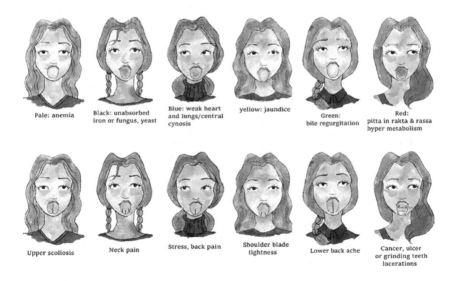

| Pale: anemia | Black: unabsorbed iron or fungus, yeast | Blue: weak heart and lungs/central cynosis | yellow: jaundice | Green: bile regurgitation | Red: pitta in rakta & rassa hyper metabolism |

| Upper scoliosis | Neck pain | Stress, back pain | Shoulder blade tightness | Lower back ache | Cancer, ulcer or grinding teeth lacerations |

Your Bowel Movements

I always ask my patients what their bowel movements look like. I often get answers such as, "I never look; I just flush," or "Yuck!" Like it or not, your stools are another feedback feature of your body. You need to be looking before you flush. Check the color, shape, size, frequency, odor, and consistency of your bowel movements. What you want to see in the toilet is a brown, banana-shaped stool that is easy to wipe after, has little odor, doesn't stick to the toilet, and is eliminated in the morning regardless of what you have eaten.

If you have mucous, blood, undigested food, dry stools, watery or loose stools, infrequent or frequent stools, this is feedback that can trigger you to search further for the cause.

Your Urine

Your urine is a product of your kidneys filtering your toxins. Your urine ought to be about 1.5 liters per day, pale yellow, infrequent, and passed without pain or urgency. If you have darker urine, you might be dehydrated. If you have cloudy urine, you could have an infection. Urine with an abnormal color or odor or accompanying pain is feedback from your body. Pay attention; you ignore it at your own risk. If you have an imbalance, it will move from one layer of tissue to another the longer it's ignored.

Your Sweat

When you exercise, you ought to sweat. Your skin is the largest organ of detoxification you have. It's important that you use it by sweating each day to rid yourself of unwanted toxins and pollutants. However, your sweat is not supposed to have a strong odor. While you might not smell like roses after a long hike, you will also not offend the people around you with your smell if you are healthy. Strong body odor can be a sign of toxicity. A lack of sweat can indicate adrenal fatigue; an abundance of perspiration means your adrenal glands are revved up too high and you are on your way to adrenal fatigue.

Your Hair and Nails

Your hair and nails are another feedback mechanism. What is normal for you will be in accord with your dosha mix. Vata hair is thinner and finer, pitta hair can have a reddish tint to it and appear wavy or curly. Kapha hair will be lustrous and thick. Anything outside of your dosha type's "normal" will be abnormal for you.

For example, when a kapha woman is in my office telling me she is losing too much hair, I need to listen even though her hair might appear thick to me. If a man comes in wanting to talk about what he considers premature balding, if he is a pitta dosha type, I need to address a potential imbalance of his dosha. Pitta people are at risk for premature greying and balding. However, male pattern baldness can also signal too much testosterone for men or women. Loss of hair that feels like straw and is dry to the touch can reflect thyroid and adrenal imbalance. Hair falling out in chunks can mean you have parasites in your gut. Greasy hair might indicate you have a kapha imbalance.

The same rule of "normal for the dosha type" is true for fingernails. Vata nails are thinner and more brittle. Pitta nails are soft and pink, and kapha nails are thick and strong.

Your fingernails ought to have a half moon at the cuticle or base of the nail on each finger. They should look and feel smooth rather than rough or ridged. White spots can indicate a zinc or calcium deficiency. Pale nails can be a red flag for anemia while a yellow nail is a sign of a liver imbalance. Blue nails usually signal heart or lung problems.

Your Skin

Skin is one of the first places an imbalance will show up. Do not ignore the signs on your skin. Each of us has skin that is typical and healthy for our dosha type. Vata people can have thinner, dryer skin prone to wrinkles as they age. Pitta folks have skin at risk for inflammation. Their skin will be more likely to have moles and freckles, burn easily and break out more readily. Kapha skin is thicker, oilier, and can be prone to cysts and boils.

Antibiotics do not treat the root cause of acne. If you have an inflammatory issue such as acne, rosacea, psoriasis, or eczema, think digestive imbalance rather than topical skin-care products. Leaky gut, or intestinal permeability, is the root cause for autoimmune disease, including autoimmune issues of the skin such as psoriasis and eczema. As we covered earlier, intestinal permeability or leaky gut is a disruption in the lining of the intestinal wall. This allows undigested food molecules to escape into the body where the immune system fights against them as if they were a virus or bacteria.

Leaky gut is the root cause for many diseases. One of the first places it shows up is on the tongue and on the skin. Pay attention to the feedback your body is giving you so it doesn't have to turn up the volume and scream to be heard.

Your Facial Lines

Hopefully this discussion serves to raise your awareness of the signs your body sends you when it's out of balance. You can go out of balance when the weather changes, if you don't get enough sleep or too much sleep, if you don't eat right for your body type, if you are having mental or emotional stress, as you age, if you don't hydrate properly, if you exercise at the wrong time of day or in a way that doesn't match your body type. Your body is constantly attempting to stay in balance, but if you don't pay attention, if might get so far out of balance that it's hard to come back. Ultimately, this can result in chronic or acute disease. *Figure 21* gives you an example of what your facial lines are telling you about your health.

▼ **Figure 21:** Ayurvedic facial mappinge tongue

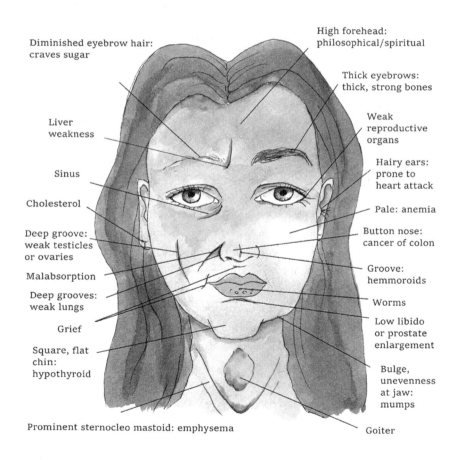

High forehead: philosophical/spiritual

Diminished eyebrow hair: craves sugar

Thick eyebrows: thick, strong bones

Liver weakness

Weak reproductive organs

Sinus

Hairy ears: prone to heart attack

Cholesterol

Pale: anemia

Deep groove: weak testicles or ovaries

Button nose: cancer of colon

Malabsorption

Groove: hemmoroids

Deep grooves: weak lungs

Worms

Grief

Low libido or prostate enlargement

Square, flat chin: hypothyroid

Bulge, unevenness at jaw: mumps

Prominent sternocleo mastoid: emphysema

Goiter

The 6 Stages of Disease Progression

As discussed in Chapter 7, Ayurvedic medicine teaches us that we have 7 tissue layers, or dhatus. Healthy tissues are created by the proper digestion of our foods, thoughts, and emotions. If you are not properly digesting or are not making nutritious choices for your individual body type, a couple of things result: First, the tissue layers will not be healthy and strong because of built-up toxicity, or ama. Second, an imbalanced dosha will move from its place of origin to a place of weakness in the body and create further imbalance.

There are 6 stages of dis-ease progression as the body becomes more and more imbalanced. The 6 stages of disease are:

- **Stage 1:** Accumulation
- **Stage 2:** Aggravation
- **Stage 3:** Dissemination
- **Stage 4:** Localization
- **Stage 5:** Manifestation
- **Stage 6:** Disruption

It is said that in our culture we do not usually notice or pay attention to our imbalance until it has progressed to full blown disease, stage 4 or 5, when our forward motion and productivity are impaired. I know this was true for me and I see it every day in my medical practice. The fast-paced, productivity-oriented society we live in has us so out of touch with our bodies and minds that we do not notice the first signs of imbalance.

Integration Exercise: Connecting to Your body

Developing a common language with your body is the first step to move from combat to collaboration with it. Remember, autoimmune disease means you are in combat with your own body, and there is no winner. Your body is the vehicle carrying you around. It's important that you know when it needs some tender loving care.

Here are some simplified self-care activities that will allow you to connect to your body. Try these at home. Take the dosha quiz (resources section) to find out your unique birth constitution. Then download more dosha-specific daily routine ideas in the WILD Program.

1. Scrape your tongue twice a day. After brushing your teeth, use a tongue scraper, a "U" shaped metal tool to scrape your tongue. Put the rounded end toward the back of your tongue and throat and pull forward 5–7 times. Note if there is a coating.

2. Look at your stools and urine before you flush the toilet.

3. Self-massage each morning and/or at night before bed. Use sesame oil if you are a vata-predominate person, coconut oil if you are pitta with inflammation, and olive or almond oil if you are kapha.

CHAPTER 9

No One Size Fits All

*"I'm a big believer in what's called personalized medi-
cine, which refers to customizing your healthcare to your
specific needs based on your physiology, genetics, value
system and unique conditions."*

~DAVID AGUS, MD

Personalizing Medicine

The Freedom Framework that I have taught you so far is the perfect tool to help you personalize your own medical care. To this point, you have learned how to frame all four sides of your puzzle and to see how the four corner pieces fit in. As a refresher, the four sides of the Freedom Framework are:

1. Un-**C**over the root causes, which will be found in:
   a. Your body.
   b. Your mind.
   c. Your emotions.
   d. Your spirit.
   e. Your story and how you tell it.

2. **C**onfront the data collected through laboratory testing and your own story.

3. **C**onnect your beliefs and behaviors with your current reality.

4. **C**reate the life you want to be living with full intention.

The four corner pieces of your puzzle are: 1) leaky gut, 2) environmental toxins, 3) genetics, and 4) trauma. After framing your puzzle, you can begin filling in the center pieces to create the picture you want to live with. You will want to heal the areas along the edges that are causing you trouble.

Healing leaky gut and detoxifying built-up accumulation of gene-altering toxicity needs to be done in a personalized way. (I teach my approach to this in the Whole Individualized Life Detox (WILD) Program.) In Chapter 10, you will learn to identify your held-onto hurts, and heal the gene-altering, toxic beliefs you have unknowingly carried with you from childhood. These are preventing you from completely healing your leaky gut and so keeping you from living with full joy, passion, and vitality.

Remember, there is no one-size-fits-all program for reversing autoimmune disease, any more than there is a specific diet right for everyone with inflammation or autoimmunity. There are general guidelines I will give you regarding food choices, but no book can give you what is absolutely true for you and your unique case. The same holds true for supplements. I use test results from each of my patients to inform my advice. Why? You now know that autoimmunity is complex and there are several different root causes that must be addressed. These will be different for everyone.

That said, everyone with autoimmunity has leaky gut and must heal their digestive system to get ahead of their immune system's hyper-reactivity. Your leaky gut might be accompanied by a gut infection, food sensitivities, toxicity, and some of the variables we have talked about already. So though the overview I gave you in Chapter 5 about healing leaky gut is a good start, you cannot heal completely unless you have addressed the other 3 corner pieces of your puzzle as well: toxins/infections, genetics, and trauma.

Test, Don't Guess

Functional medicine testing is different from the Uncle SAM model of testing. When you have an autoimmune disease, your body produces antibodies against your own tissues. Diagnosing an autoimmune disease involves identifying the antibodies your body is producing. However, remember, it can take several decades to develop an autoimmune disease. It's important to be on the watch for signs your health is about to go over a cliff so you can turn it around in time. It is much easier to prevent autoimmunity or to reverse an autoimmune disease in the early stages than it is in later stages when organ damage has already occurred.

The following tests are used in the standard American medical model to diagnose autoimmunity:

- Autoantibody tests: any of several tests that look for specific antibodies to your own tissues.

- Antinuclear antibody tests: a type of autoantibody test that looks for anti-nuclear antibodies, which attack the nuclei of cells in your body.

- Complete blood count: measures the numbers of red and white cells in your blood. When your immune system is actively fighting something, these numbers will vary from the normal.

- C-reactive protein (CRP): elevated CRP is an indication of inflammation throughout your body.

- Erythrocyte sedimentation rate: this test indirectly measures how much inflammation is in your body.

Functional Medicine Lab Tests for Getting to the Root Cause(s)

Now that you know you are your own health advocate, you will no longer expect your insurance company to pay for prevention, right? It would sure be nice if it would, but the reality of our current healthcare system is that health insurance is not the same as health assurance. So the likelihood is that your insurance won't cover all of the costs of reversing your autoimmune disease. Expect to pay at least some out-of-pocket costs for the appropriate testing.

The following tests give me data that allows me to help my patients solve the autoimmune puzzle at the root cause level rather than surface symptom management:

- Thyroid Panel (blood): TSH, Free T3, Free T4, RT3, TPO Ab, Tg Ab, TR Ab, TSHR Ab, TSI

- Inflammatory Panel (blood): Sed rate, HS CRP, Homocysteine

- Blood sugar metabolism panel (blood): Hgb A1c, insulin, fasting blood sugar

- Liver and Kidneys (blood): chem panel, MTHFR, and GGT

- Lipids (blood): Total cholesterol, LDL, HDL, TGL, size, density, particle count, LPa, PLAC, APOB, APOE

- Vitamin D3 (blood)

- Hormone Panel (blood): fractionated estrogens, progesterone, free and total testosterone, sex hormone binding globulin, FSH, LH, DHEAs, and PSA if male

- CBC with diff

- Food sensitivity/allergy panel (blood): IgG and IgE
- Adrenal and Hormone Panel (saliva): cortisol x 4, fractionated estrogen, progesterone, testosterone, melatonin, DHEA, pregnelonone
- Comprehensive Stool Analysis (stool): enzymes, fat absorption, inflammation, sIgA, parasites, yeast, H. Pylori, bacterial over growth in the small intestines (SIBO)
- SIBO Breath test
- Urine Organics
- Heavy metal testing pre- and post-provocation (urine)
- Hormone metabolism (urine)
- Micronutrient and fatty acid profile testing (urine, blood)
- Genetics (saliva)

Before testing, I listen to the story of my client to ascertain which tests to run and choose them on an as-needed basis. All of these tests are not necessary for most people and are never necessary all at the same time.

Again, most functional medicine testing is not covered by insurance plans. The data that comes from these tests is not connected to the pharmaceutical industry, and the results will reveal imbalances that can be rectified by diet, lifestyle changes, and targeted nutritional supplementation.

Heal Emotional Wounds

There are hundreds of thousands of toxins, outside of the ones we have already discussed, that pollute your brain every year. I'm talking about the thoughts and feelings that make you feel fearful, anxious, guilty, or ashamed. Yes, these too are toxins and mess with your immune system and hormone levels.

Your thoughts and feelings are digested by your mind and heart much the same way food is digested by your digestive system. What you get from food is nourishment that gives you energy, vitality, and continued life as you create new cells from nutrients. What do you get from your thoughts and feelings? First you have a feeling, then a thought, and then you take action. So nourishing thoughts and feelings generate vitality-building actions. As food provides nourishment to create new cells, healthy thoughts and feelings generate actions that "create" your life.

Painful feelings and thoughts, on the other hand, are held in the body if they are not processed well. Early painful experiences can leave a "button" exposed for others to push later. If someone or something pushes that button, it can trigger the hormone cascade that begins in the brain when you believe you are in danger or under attack. If this happens too often, your body will begin to believe you are that zebra being chased by a lion we talked about earlier, and in danger of being eaten. Your hormones will respond by sending the stress hormone cortisol out into your bloodstream so you can have the energy to run from the lion or turn and fight it.

The problem is that there is not really a lion behind you and all of that cortisol breaks down your gut wall and starts making your body store fat. Eventually your body just holds onto weight because it feels like it's constantly in danger and wants to make sure you have enough nutrients on board in case you can't stop to eat. Eventually you will start having your progesterone supplies reallocated to the adrenal glands to keep you in survival mode. The resulting estrogen dominance puts you at risk for breast cancer, autoimmune disease, as well as moodiness and weight gain.

Unless you consciously change how you perceive and react to stress in your life, you will continue in the same pattern. It takes conscious awareness to change the patterns you have been repeating throughout your life, and often it takes psychotherapy.

There are many thoughts, beliefs, and feelings that can create a hypervigilant immune system and play havoc with the hormones in your body. In fact, this is where we can be the least free…in our minds. Below I list 7 feelings that are present in people with an autoimmune mindset, but spend some time thinking of others that might be keeping you stuck. We will explore this more in the next chapter.

Shame

Shame is an emotion that is a sure vitality sucker. You are not capable of feeling love and shame at the same time. Shame creates contraction in your body and love is experienced as openness.

Try this: If you are feeling shame, find a moment in your life that you have felt love and spend time with that thought instead of the one causing you pain.

Hate

Hate usually arises because someone has betrayed or hurt you deeply. This is not a feeling that goes with feeling fabulous. The way out of hate is forgiveness. You have likely heard this before and are rolling your eyes right now. But let me just stop you before you quit reading here. I am not saying you have to reconcile with anyone who has caused you harm. I believe in having healthy boundaries with toxic people.

Try this: Think of the personality trait the person who hurt you exhibited that you really hate. Is it selfishness? Is it cruelty? Is it misusing power? How about a lack of integrity? Write in your journal any and all of the ego characteristics you find in the person you are focusing on right now.

Next look at them in the heart as if you are looking in the mirror. They are only reflecting the very human personality traits that you, me, and everyone else on this planet have. We all have the same traits! It's true. We just do them differently, so it looks like we are so very different from the one we hate.

For example: Adolf Hitler could be said to have misused power and been cruel. I can say that I have done both of those things (maybe even before breakfast today because I'm a mom and have to really watch not using the old guilt treatment on my teenager). I have never bought tanks and taken over Poland. I have never killed anyone. I will never do those things… BUT I have manifested two of the personality traits I identify in Hitler.

Make sense? Try it yourself. Go deep and don't be afraid to look at what triggers you. You do it too…just differently than the one you hate.

This leads to forgiveness. When you are no longer blaming, judging, hating the other person, you can more readily forgive.

Remember what Mark Twain said so eloquently, "Not forgiving is like you drinking poison and expecting the other guy to die." Or the Chinese proverb that says, "Don't forgive…dig two graves instead of one."

Perfection

I cannot tell you how many people I have worked with in therapy that are trapped by the perfection myth. That you have to be perfect to be worthy of love is something you decided when you were a small child in response to events you didn't know how to process differently. This one is a cage that you will never heal in. You are worthy of love just by virtue of being who you are…a gift to this world with your own unique talents and skills you bring. You are perfect just as you are.

Try this: Go pick up that little girl or boy inside you and let him or her know just how much YOU love her. Let her know she doesn't have to DO anything for you to love her. She just has to be herself, and you will support and adore her no matter what. Forgive yourself for thinking anything else. You won't heal without doing this.

Safety

How can you possibly relax if you do not feel safe? If you are truly unsafe, then make the necessary changes to make yourself safe. Every woman deserves to live free. Unfortunately, many in our world do not. If you are reading this, you are likely in a position to create safety in your life if you set your mind and will to it.

Not feeling safe is a result of a childhood trauma, stressor, or experience you did not have the skills to process. You likely had good reason to feel unsafe. Ask yourself now if it's still true that you are not safe. What triggers that feeling in you today? Is it a big red button that you are hyper-vigilant about? Is it pressed all too easily? If so it is a good idea to get some work with a trained EMDR therapist or a therapist who is certified in Brainspotting or clinical hypnotherapy.

A zebra being chased by a lion is not going to feel safe. Are you a zebra? Is your libido gone? Do you have bowel issues? Are your hormones imbalanced? Do you have autoimmune disease? Feeling unsafe plays havoc on your entire hormone system and can lead to obesity, fatigue, sleeplessness, low sexual desire, PMS, hot flashes, vaginal dryness, memory issues, brain fog, autoimmunity, and more.

Try this: The next time you are triggered by someone who leaves you feeling abandoned, unsafe, lonely, or hurt, close your eyes. Take a deep breath and really feel where the feeling of danger lives in your body.

Is it in your shoulders? In your gut? In your throat or jaw or chest? Now ask yourself how old you feel. Are you very, very young?

Go get that little one and give her a big hug and reassure her that whatever she experienced as a child is not going to happen again because you are watching over her and keeping her safe. Bring her into your heart and love her. Feel how safe you both are. Breathe that feeling of grounded safety into the areas of tension in your body. Do this until you are relaxed again.

Emotional Freedom Technique, or "tapping" is another tool for reducing the feelings of overwhelm that can occur when you don't feel safe. There is a video in the resource section that you can use to learn EFT. Practice it often so it becomes second nature to use when you are feeling unsafe.

Not Enough

Scarcity complex is an insidious trap that haunts you if you have thoughts of "not enough time," "not enough friends," "not enough energy," "not enough money" not enough connection with my partner," "not enough...."

Try this: Write a positive affirmation that affirms your abundance. Whatever we spend time thinking about comes true, so make sure it's something you want to manifest. For example: "I easily and effortlessly attract abundance of all kinds into my life. I am grateful for all of the love, resources, time, and energy I possess."

I Will Be Happy When...

This is a black hole if there ever was one. It leads straight to feeling stuck.

Have you ever caught yourself thinking, "I will be happy when I lose weight," or "I will be happy when I have a boyfriend, or a partner, or get married," or "I will be happy when I can finally pay off my bills, or get that promotion"? You get the idea. My guess is every human being has done this.

Try this: Find all of the things in your life you can be grateful for. Gratitude is powerful medicine and puts you on the road to feeling fabulous fast. Keeping a gratitude journal is a wonderful daily practice. We all have something to feel grateful for, but we often lose sight of those things because our stressors seem to fill our viewing screen.

When you wake up in the morning, begin with expressing gratitude for the very fact that you woke up. Then start listing even the smallest things you can think of. They all add up to an infinite number of blessings to be grateful for.

- Did you wake up in a bed with a roof over your head?

- Are you getting out of bed and stepping on two feet that can still carry you around?

- Are you about to brush teeth that you have to chew your food with?

- Can you see with your eyes to know where to go?

So many blessings and so little time to express thanks for them. When you fill your mind with thoughts of appreciation, it fosters love, and that makes everyone feel fabulous.

I Can't

Self-limiting beliefs are your biggest enemy, not sugar, and I consider sugar one of the biggest toxins there is. But when it comes to inflammation and toxicity, by far self-limiting beliefs trump sugar.

Self-limiting beliefs keep you caged. You are not free to live to your highest potential. The worst part of this is you are doing it to yourself. If you ever hear yourself think or say, "I can't _____ (fill in the blank)" then STOP. Realize you just put yourself in a cage of your own making.

Try this: I am challenging you to say "I can" whenever you get the chance. Does this mean you say yes to everyone who wants you to volunteer for their organization? Does it mean you over schedule yourself so your own self-care goes out the window? No. You get to tell people no. You get to set healthy boundaries for yourself and with yourself.

It does mean you say "I can" when you want to try something new that may be a stretch. It means you go beyond your self-imposed limits. Make this the week of "I can." Then make it a month of "I can." Then try a year of "I can." Yeah! By then you will be on your way to a lifetime of accepting the opportunities the Universe puts in your path for your growth and for unfolding your potential.

Supplementation

Now that you have learned how to supplant nourishing beliefs with toxic ones, let's move onto nutritional supplementation. As I have said, there is no single appropriate supplement program for everyone with autoimmune disease. There is no one supplement program for every woman. However, there are some general supplementation guidelines that will start you on your journey to healing.

First, not all supplements with the same name are of the same quality. In the realm of nutritional supplements, you really do get what you pay for. The companies that take the time to test for quality, toxins, and purity are the companies I recommend. Going to a big box store will save you money in the short term, but studies have shown that what is on the label is not what is in the bottle. Every study that has been done to evaluate supplement quality has discovered that discount supplement brands are cutting corners and giving the rest of the industry a bad name.

Second, your body's ability to digest and absorb nutrients and then eliminate toxins is going to affect how well you react to supplementation. If you are not absorbing nutrients from food, it will be difficult for you to absorb multiple supplements. This is why testing is so important as you embark on your autoimmune reversal journey.

Third, make sure your supplements (and medications if you take them) do not contain gluten, dairy, artificial colors and preservatives, binders and bulkers, or sugar. Gelatin, mannitol, xylitol, dextrin, and magnesium stearate are considered safe.

There are eight supplements I recommend to everyone with leaky gut and autoimmune disease. They can be taken according to the label instructions and adjusted depending on lab results. The brand I have vetted many times over is called Functional Nutrients. They are of the highest quality and are very effective, plus they are the ones I use in my practice.

1. **L-Glutamine:** Glutamine is an amino acid the intestines use to rebuild and repair damage. It helps heal leaky gut by protecting the gut wall from further damage. It's also a neurotransmitter, or brain chemical, that helps with focus, concentration, and memory. It helps your cells get rid of toxins and helps curb sugar cravings. As with every supplement and herb, sometimes L-Glutamine will react poorly with some people. Always stop any supplement that creates a negative reaction and check with your medical provider.

2. **Fish oil:** EPA and DHA, which are ingredients in fish oil, are not only anti-inflammatory, but they help with healthy gene expression. It is imperative that you choose a brand, such as Functional Nutrients, that has undergone voluntary toxicity testing. We have polluted our oceans to such a degree that the fish we are obtaining our fish oil from are often toxic.

   You might have read about the health benefits of krill oil. Please do not use krill oil. Krill are tiny sea creatures that are the primary diet of some of the largest life forms on our planet, baleen whales, like the blue and humpback whales. These magnificent creatures do not have the multitudes of choices for their diets like humans do. We can get our oil from small fish from the sea that are at low risk for the toxic burden that large fish such as salmon now have. Krill also play a huge role in absorbing carbon from the atmosphere. For these reasons and more, we need to ensure that the krill population does not continue its alarming decline.

3. **Probiotics:** Probiotics are important for strengthening your gut's microbiome. Supporting your microbiome is key in reversing disease, attaining a healthy weight, and maintaining hormone balance. Probiotics help you live a life that includes joy, a good memory, and a healthy libido. I recommend a probiotic with a strong diversity and large number of colony-forming units.

Before we ever had probiotics in bottles, we had fermented foods. Our ancestors kept their digestive health strong by eating the ferment that was popular in their culture. Eating a variety of ferments such as sauerkraut and coconut milk kefir will give you microbes produced by these very different fermented products. Korean kimchee will provide a different strain of microbes than Peruvian chicha will. Diversity is important as you are aiming for a strong and healthy collaborative ecosystem in your gut. However, certain genetic SNPs do not support the high tyramine content contained in fermented foods and bone broth.

4. **Vitamin D3:** Vitamin D is a key player in the health of the junctions between the cells of your gut wall. You want your junctions to be tight, so food and toxins cannot escape through your gut wall and into your bloodstream. Autoimmune diseases, such as multiple sclerosis, occur at higher rates in areas that do not get consistent sunlight. The low levels of vitamin D that result from low sun exposure impact the gut wall by loosening the junctions between the cells in the lining. Ask your medical provider to check your vitamin D level every 6 months and make sure your levels are consistently between 70 ng/mL and 90 ng/mL.

5. **Immuno Gut:** Immuno Gut is an egg-derived immunoglobulin. It's been shown to be effective against 26 different human pathogens including strep, e coli, salmonella, staph, and more. It's also effective for gut healing, SIBO, autoimmunity, cardiovascular health, and systemic inflammation.

6. **InflammaCore:** InflammaCore contains herbs and nutrients for reducing inflammation, tissue damage, and aiding in lymphatic drain-

age: Boswellia, ginger, quercetin, rutin, rosemary, and resveratrol.

7. **Immuno-Mod:** Immuno-Mod contains ingredients such as curcumin, which have been shown to reduce inflammation and modulate how the immune system responds to perceived triggers.

8. **Collagen:** HSN Complex is one of my favorite supplements to take personally. The collagen in HSN Complex aids in healing the gut wall, healthy skin, hormone balance, thick hair and strong nails, as well as in cellulite removal. Another way of getting collagen every day is to drink ½ cup of bone broth. I have provided you with my favorite recipe for bone broth. I make it and drink it during the cold months of the year. This recipe is delicious.

WILD Program

It has been my experience that people are more successful in creating new habits when they tell others what they are up to, ask for support, and make changes with a community of people who are on the same path and willing to act as accountability partners for one another. It's likely this book does not contain everything you will need to make a significant life transformation for your particular case. If I included every detail required for every person to adjust every single piece of their individual puzzle, the book would be longer than the Bible and near impossible to apply.

I do, however, have a program that you can begin after finishing the book. It's the next step. It's called the Whole Individualized Life Detox (WILD) Program and it's 5 modules that are online that you can take along with thousands of other women who are taking it. You will all get to "meet" and "know" each other in the private WILD Program online group. There you will be able to take quizzes that help you identify how to individualize your healing program. You will get meal plans, recipes, a guide for following the SCD diet, video demonstrations, emotional healing tools, audio meditations, tracking tools, supplement protocols, and testing and private coaching options. The WILD Program is designed to give you Wellness, Information, Love, and Detoxification at the pace you can manage them.

Becoming a WILD Woman

The WILD Program is in alignment with my wish to help you become a

WILD woman, or a woman who is living as naturally and close to the earth and heaven as she can. A WILD woman is not caged by her mind traps or stuck in a vicious cycle of disease. She is willing, eager, and motivated to make the changes she needs to be the brightest, strongest version of herself. She runs with a pack of other WILD women and knows that her presence in the tribe is not only a glorious gift to all that she is in community with, but is necessary for the strength of the whole group.

A WILD woman is keenly aware of and trusts her intuition. She works tirelessly on integrating the insights gained from the inevitable hurt that comes to her in life. She is in communication with her mind, her heart, her body, and her spirit and moves sometimes gracefully through her life cycles and sometimes stumbles. When she is stuck, she asks for help. When she sees one who is stuck, she provides compassionate wisdom. She forgives herself for the hurts she has held onto; she forgives those who have hurt her, and she forgives herself for the hurts she has inflicted.

She sets healthy boundaries. She howls at the moon when she needs to, and she smiles serenely when she wants to. She expresses her feelings and is willing to alter her beliefs when she sees that it is time to expand into a new level of consciousness. She sings, she dances, she creates; she is sensual and she is sexual. She loves, she cries, she accepts what she cannot change, she surrenders what she cannot control, she grows, she expands, she learns, she laughs, and she lives fully. A WILD woman is a goddess.

You are a goddess. Do you always remember that you are part of the brilliance of this Universe? Do you know how essential you are? If not, you are likely stuck in some old patterns of hurt that have created self-limiting beliefs keeping you from feeling your divine nature. Chapter 10 is the big chapter. It's the chapter that dives deeply into finding and healing your old HURT. It's the secret sauce. It's the magic. It's the good stuff and the hard stuff. Return to it again and again and work through it layer by layer. Old HURT is not bad. Those old childhood experiences that caused pain are the places that you mine your wisdom from. This is where the gold is.

CHAPTER 10

Finding Your HURT

"Healing is a matter of time, but it is sometimes also a matter of opportunity."

~HIPPOCRATES

While traveling in Kashmir, India, I was told the creation story of the beautiful Kashmir diamond. The ibex is a kind of wild goat found in the mountains of Ladakh and Baltistan. They spend the warm days of summer atop the most inaccessible places, usually cliffs, descending only to graze. The ibex is a cautious animal, careful to avoid being harmed. Before descending from the cliffs, an older buck is put on sentry duty on a prominent rock to keep watch over the grazing herd. It is said that the sentry ibex kills and eats venomous snakes when he encounters them. As the venom enters his bloodstream, he falls asleep on the hot stones of the cliff. The highly acidic venom leaks from his mouth as he sleeps, onto the hot rocks, where it eats through the stone, forming fissures. As the day wanes and the temperature changes, the fissures close. This creates the chemistry that eventually forms a Kashmir diamond. These rare gems find their way to the marketplace through local gem dealers who occasionally receive the precious stones from goat herders who find them in the cliffs. They are considered to be of great value for their beauty, scarcity, and quality.

The point of this legend for us is that releasing the inner hurt left over from painful experiences and trauma brings a priceless reward, more precious than diamonds. And what is that? Freedom. Freedom from autoimmune disease. Freedom to live a life infused with health and vitality. Conversely, a rigid mind full of resentment, victimhood, bitterness, and venom creates a rigid body with an immune system that stays on the attack.

Part of being human means you will be hurt, and you will perpetrate hurt. Being traumatized is part of life on earth. Healing that hurt is what leads to compassion, wisdom, and freedom from disease. You are going to learn a beautiful exercise that will help you release the need to hold onto your past hurt. You are going to learn how to reverse the autoimmune mindset of judgement, expectations, and blame. This process is how you are going to attain freedom from inflammation and how you will alter the interior of your puzzle.

I often hear from my patients with autoimmune disease that they have never had trauma. This is untrue. Every human has had traumatic experiences. Bringing them to your awareness is not dwelling on them or rehashing them. It's the place you start to really process them with your adult brain. In the last chapter I introduced you to examples of toxic thoughts that keep leaky gut from healing, upregulate genes that can lead to disease, and are a result of early painful experiences. You learned how to change those toxic thoughts to nourishing ones. Now let's take a deeper look at the role emotional wounds play in autoimmunity.

Identifying Your HURT

In 2012, I conducted a pilot study called the HURT (Healing Un-Resolved Trauma) study. I interviewed 89 American women ages 27 to 76 years of age. I asked them if there was a correlation between past emotional hurts and present-day low libido. The results of the study indicated that yes, past hurt in childhood creates a button that can then be pushed by people later in your life. When this happens, it activates the 4F stress response system that results in high blood pressure, an increase in heart rate, diminished libido, and a dysfunctional immune system. I also found that healing the trauma, learning to forgive, and the willingness to self-confront patterns of reactivity could reverse not only low libido, but inflammation and disease too. It was a matter of retraining and reframing (*see figure 22*).

A Dog Chases Its Tail and the Mind Chases Its Tale

Now here's the catch when it comes to retraining yourself: When you perceive there is a problem and ask the very same mind that created the problem, through its own perceptions, to solve the problem, you are creating a "dog chasing its tail" scenario. Except in this case, your mind is chasing its tale...

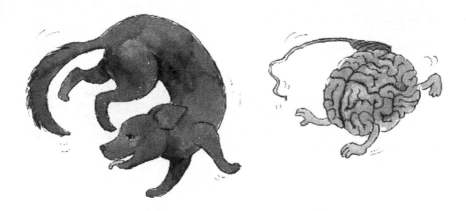

The solution to this lies in the difference between *adaptive* memory processing and *maladaptive* memory looping. Maladaptive looping is ruminating on ANTs (automatic negative thoughts) that emerge from feeling hurt, betrayed, unsafe, unworthy, unlovable, unheard, unseen, unimportant, not good enough, and so on. With adaptive memory processing, you stop chasing this belief, or tale. You tire of triggering over the same hurts again and again. You see repeated patterns in your life and realize your reactions to them are not serving you or those around you. To get your mind to stop chasing its tale, you must be willing to self-confront, to work with the story you have written, and to rewrite it. If you are not willing, you will not be free. It's that simple. The Freedom Framework is about getting unstuck. It's about letting go of patterns that keep you looping and loopy. It's about releasing pain of all kinds because you are tired of being in pain. It's about being free of autoimmune disease.

The HURT
(Healing Un-Resolved Trauma) Model

"Ignore those that make you fearful and sad, that degrade you back towards disease and death."

~RUMI

Let's walk through the HURT model using my story so you can see how this works. Please refer to the HURT Model diagram to follow along (*see figure 22*).

▼ **Figure 22**

The HURT (Healing Un-Resolved Trauma) Modelease

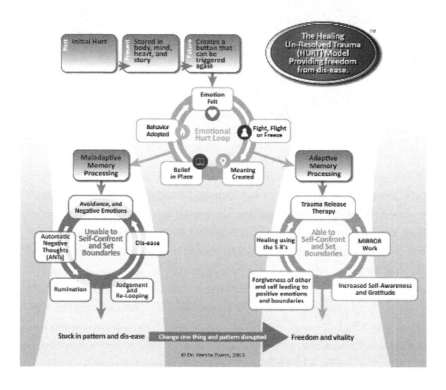

1. **Initial hurt from the past:** I will use my sexual abuse at age 10 as the initial event.

2. **The hurt is stored in the body, mind, heart, and story:** Clearly this was distressing for my little girl-self on all levels: physical, mental, emotional, spiritual, and it became a pivotal part of my story. I had plenty of evidence to create the beliefs or tales that I was still carrying when I was diagnosed with rheumatoid arthritis: "The world is not safe, people in authority are not safe, and therefore I am not safe," "I have to be perfect or I won't survive," "When the going gets tough, I can check out." This last belief reflected the times in my life that I had fantasized about dying and being in a "better place" where there were angels, loving deceased family members, and no one violated little girls. When things got too dark in my head, the light would go out. I just wanted to die. Autoimmunity was the agreement my cells had made with this message.

3. **A button was created that can be triggered in the future:** Whenever I felt unsafe or rejected, I would do anything in my power to make it right. I was a people pleaser and rescuer. I set up co-dependent relationships to help me feel worthy of being on the earth. It was part of my survival mechanism. The problem with this, and all other childhood strategies that rely on outside approval for self-worth, is it's impossible to please everyone. It's impossible to make everyone like you. Co-dependency is a roller coaster of emotional slavery. It does not lead to self-differentiation or an empowered sense of self.

4. **Emotion felt:** When I felt unsafe, anxious, and powerless as a child, I usually felt it in my gut and heart. Later, when I went through yoga teacher training, my teacher could tell that I had a history of trauma. Why? Because my shoulders caved forward, to protect my heart she said. I will have those slightly stooped shoulders for the rest of my life. They are a reminder to me to make sure my heart is open and vulnerable. I also developed leaky gut. I will also need to be aware of my digestive system for the rest of my life, treating it with tender loving care.

5. **Activation of fight, flight, faint, or freeze (4F stress response system):** Anyone who didn't like me, said terrible things about me, stopped talking to me, got angry at me, and so on, could set off the primal response in my brain that screamed "danger" to the rest of my body. The stress hormone cortisol was then released so I could flee or fight my danger. However, there is nothing to run away from, so the cortisol remained in my system, triggering my heart rate to increase, my bowels to shut down, and my weight to go up. I had constipation for years. Because this happened over and over again, the cortisol began to break down the lining on the inside of my intestinal wall, which contributed to leaky gut.

6. **Meaning created:** The meaning that I created in my undeveloped and immature mind was the world is unsafe and I am unimportant. If I were important, someone would protect me from harm.

7. **Belief in place:** The belief I created was that I had to be perfect to be safe and to survive this life. It was an administrator in my elementary school who molested me. I was called to the office at random times during the week from class. I believed if I was absolutely perfect and well-behaved, perhaps these distressing calls would cease.

8. **Behavior adopted:** I became adept at reading the signals of an unhappy parent, adults in authority, and other kids. I have found that the more adverse childhood experiences a person has had, the more intuitive they are. Just ask any psychic about their childhood. That intuitive radar was highly developed at an early age.

I did everything I could to "fix" conflict. I also tried hard to be "perfect" so as not to get into trouble and be abandoned or rejected. I learned to make myself useful and indispensable. Caregiving was my strategy for survival. Look what I do for a living now. This is no accident.

Now that the button is in place, created in my childhood, it can be triggered by anyone who comes along who I perceive is rejecting me or threatening me or my family. This button has wires that connect to my brain, my heart, and my immune system. If I didn't confront this maladaptive processing loop created in my childhood, this button could and would be triggered by anyone who comes along the rest of my life. It's like a time bomb, ready to go off every time the wire is tripped inadvertently by a passersby. The very same cascade of reactions I experienced in childhood will be repeated at potentially the same scale as they were in the past.

A lifetime of this pattern leads not only to leaky gut and intense food and chemical intolerances, but also causes my genetics to express in ways that lead to autoimmune disease and cancer. In short, I was becoming intolerant to my own life. When I was diagnosed with RA, I had a choice, a fork in the road of my life as revealed by the HURT Model. I had to choose between:

- The maladaptive continual looping, which leads to dis-ease and staying stuck and loopy.
- Or the adaptive memory processing that leads to freedom through the willingness to self-confront.

Thankfully, I chose the latter and have been not only willing, but excited to self-confront my triggers. I did not want to continue down the same road of disease I was already on. It has created true freedom physically, emotionally, mentally, and spiritually.

The HURT Model Main Points

- Experiences that hurt, such as ACEs, are <u>felt</u> in the body as emotion.
- Your 4F stress response system is activated when you feel threatened.

- You make up meanings to explain the disturbing experiences from a child's perspective.
- This creates your belief structure about yourself and your world and the people you share it with.
- Behaviors are then constructed to match your beliefs and you adapt in the most skillful way you can think of with your undeveloped child brain.
- As a child, you embed this experience in your story as a factory default setting, rather than with intention.
- This creates a button that can be triggered again and again for the rest of your life. A time bomb of default settings, created by your underdeveloped brain.
- Now, as an adult, you get the amazing opportunity to upgrade your default settings.

Integration Exercise: Confronting Your HURT

The HURT Model is a pathway to freedom from held-onto hurts of all kinds. All of us have lived through the cascade of reactivity outlined in the HURT Model. Everyone has trauma in childhood. There are no exceptions, just varying degrees.

Use a journal and work through the top part of the HURT model for yourself. Recall a past hurt you experienced. This does not need to be a huge trauma. Every child experiences hurt. It's a universal human experience.

Here's an example I tell from my daughter's childhood. One day I had just gotten home from the hospital. I was still dressed in my scrubs and was greeted at the door by my young daughter. She held out her hand to me and asked me to take a splinter out of her finger. I told her I would be happy to do so. I pulled an alcohol swab and safety pin from my pocket and had her sit down. As I pulled her finger toward me, she began to cry in anticipation of the coming pain. I looked up and saw her big brown saucer shaped eyes full of terror. I quickly removed the splinter and then pulled her into my lap, rocking her and soothing her and telling her how much I loved her. What she didn't know was how happy I was in that moment.

You see, before coming home to my daughter with the tiny little splinter in her finger, I had been caring for a small toddler in the intensive care unit of the hospital I worked at in Texas. This little girl was bald, missing half of an arm, and just laid in her crib, uncomplaining. That afternoon I had inserted an intravenous solution into a vein in her scalp, a common place to access the circulatory system in babies. She had not so much as flinched when I stuck her with the large gauge needle required for her treatment. She was so used to pain, to intrusive and invasive assaults on her body, and to having people like me all around her, that she didn't even react anymore. My heart had broken for her and her family.

When I got home to my healthy daughter, full of vitality and vigor, wailing at the top of her lungs before the needle had even touched her nerve endings, I was thankful. I was grateful that this was her trauma. This was the worst thing she had experienced in her life to this point. I sent a prayer of thanks to God and loved her and cuddled her on my lap until she was soothed and ready to go play again.

Your hurt will be your hurt. It might be unresolved trauma that is abuse, or it might be a life stressor that was your worst experience. I once did hypnotherapy and trauma release for a woman whose "trauma" was always having to wear her sister's hand-me-down clothes. She had made up a meaning that she was of no value; that's why she didn't deserve anything new or nice. This was her belief. As a result, she overspent as an adult. This was her behavior. She was in severe credit card debt and trying to heal her shopping addiction. As you can see, changing the behavior is not possible without first getting to the root of the meaning and belief that drive the behavior.

1. Briefly write a hurt down. How old were you? Who was present? What happened?

_____

_____

_____

_____

_____

_____

_____

_____

_____

2. What emotion do you feel as you recount this experience?

_____

_____

_____

_____

_____

_____

_____

_____

3. What do you feel in your body? Where do you feel the emotion in your body?

_____

_____

_____

_____

_____

_____

_____

_____

4. What meaning did you create to explain the hurtful experience?

_____

_____

_____

_____

_____

_____

_____

5. What belief did you construct about yourself?

_____

_____

6. What behavior did you adopt to adapt to the meaning and belief?

7. How did this become part of your story? How do you tell this part of your story today?

8. Have you noticed this pattern repeat as this button gets pushed? What triggers it? Who triggers it?

_____

_____

_____

_____

_____

_____

_____

_____

9. Are you ready and willing to break free of this pattern?

_____

_____

_____

_____

_____

_____

_____

_____

Becoming Aware of the Mind

The mind is where you create your meanings. It's where you form your beliefs, as a result of those meanings. And from the beliefs you have formed, you adopt behaviors that are adaptive strategies in childhood, but might not work for you as an adult. With your adult brain, you now have the opportunity to become aware of the strategies you created in childhood and evaluate their efficacy in your present-day life.

This is developing what is called an observer's mind. Your higher Self can observe what your childhood ego is doing and choose to transform your behaviors, or keep them if they are nourishing you. The following integration exercises are tools I have developed over the years to help myself and my patients learn to observe ourselves, to develop self-awareness so we can take responsibility for our lives. The following exercises are to help you break the "dog chasing its tail and mind chasing its tale" cycle.

Watch Your Language

One of the most powerful tools I can give you is this simple exercise. I find that people often speak to themselves in a tone or use language that they would never use with anyone else. So for the next 24 hours observe your language. I am not concerned about profanity, grammar, or syntax in your spoken word with others in your life. I am more interested in how you speak to yourself.

Picture yourself as a small child. If you are a mother, picture one of your children when they were young. Recall in your mind an instance when your parent or another caregiver yelled at you, put you down, humiliated you, or spoke to you in a way that caused you to feel shame. Remember how deflated you felt. Think of a time when you have spoken to your own child in a way that you regretted later. Remember the look in their eyes of sadness and pain.

This is how that small child part of you feels when you speak to her in this way. You are not a fully matured woman with no past. You are a compilation of all the seconds, minutes, hours, and years you have lived. Each stage and each age is still in you. And all those aspects of you are still listening, still seeking approval, and still wanting to be loved, respected, and accepted—*especially* by you. If you cannot speak to yourself in a way that is loving, compassionate, nurturing, and respectful, why would you expect others to? If you do not give yourself this very basic human need, you are more likely to allow others to treat you as less than the powerful and beautiful goddess you are.

The next 24 hours start now, in this minute. Begin observing your language, your tone and the content of what you say to yourself. Each time you put yourself down, speak in a denigrating way to yourself, or shame yourself, I want you to push the "cancel, clear, delete" keys on your mental keyboard and replace whatever you just said with something life-affirming and positive. Maybe you made a mistake, you were at fault for something big, you really messed up, you hurt someone badly. That's okay. You can debrief this huge screw up and take what you need to know from it, so you do a better job next time. You can do all of that without berating yourself.

When a child spills his drink or breaks her glass, an attuned parent does not yell, demean, or otherwise humiliate the child. This will teach a child nothing except that it's dangerous to make a mistake. Were you that child? Do you live with the idea that it's dangerous to make a mistake? It's up to you to allow your inner child to heal from that belief. You can be the kind, wise, attuned adult for yourself that you may not have consistently had, or ever had, in childhood.

Expectations

All unhappiness comes from unmet expectations.

Your ideas about what entails a "good day" or a "bad day" are yours alone, based on meanings you have created. The value you place on the actions of others, the food you eat, your own body, and even other people are put there by you, based on meanings you have created. From your meanings and values, you create expectations. When those expectations are not met, you suffer. The more unmet expectations, the more suffering.

A Lesson from My Daughter

I have four children. When my third child was born and still very young, I was up in the middle of the night feeding her. I remember this experience so clearly. The rocking chair I used for her feedings was under a large window. That night the moon was full and cast a soft light over both of us. I could see her face clearly as she grasped my robe with one small hand and my side with another tiny hand and peacefully drew her sustenance from my breast as she nursed. Now and then she erupted with eager smiles and delightful gurgles. I was filled with the most astonishing and almost unbearable love as I gazed at this innocent infant girl who was so good natured and seemingly happy to be on planet earth.

As I rocked her, I thought about the leaders of each of the countries across the world. *If only the people who started wars and led young people into battle had the opportunity to bear and feed babies, they wouldn't be so eager to send them into battle,* I thought. I continued to feel the warm love and allowed my nurturing train of thought to continue along its rails. Then suddenly, a thought hit me: My mother had probably felt like this about me, too! Mind you I had three children at this point, and this was the first time this had occurred to me (slow learner you might say).

During my teen years, my mother and I had not gotten along well. In fact, we didn't really connect on any subject and seemed to be at odds at every turn. I had left home at 18 with her breathing a deep and palpable sigh of relief that I was gone and on my own. As an adult, visits to my parents' home were always cut short—by them. It seemed that being around my family caused them stress; it wasn't relaxing for any of us. As I rocked my baby daughter that night, I mulled these thoughts around in my head. I realized that I had a crystal-clear idea about what a mother "should be" and a father "should be" and my parents didn't match that Norman Rockwell painting in my head.

I started thinking about other people from my past that I had experienced tension with. Yep, the common thread in each of these pictures was… me. In fact, my expectations of how people "should" act had gotten in my way several times in my life. As I did this life review, it occurred to me that I had frozen my mother in time. For me, she was still the mother of my 15-year-old self. I had not let her grow in my mind as I had grown. I knew that the same was true on her side. I was stuck in her head as a stubborn 15-year-old adolescent trying to gain autonomy against tightly held reins.

How could I make sure this little daughter of mine and I stayed in harmony with one another? I vowed in that moment, in the moonlight, that I would not have expectations of her that she could not meet. Her life was her own. She was not an extension, or a reflection of me. She was her own person. I had brought her into the world, and I would raise her with love and compassion. She would have to take it from there. I am happy to say that this formula worked for all four of my children. They went through their teen years and young adult years remaining in good relationship with their father and me.

What does this have to do with autoimmune disease? Everything. If I had created expectations of my kids before they were even born, and they didn't live accordingly, I would be unhappy. I would suffer. That is the lesson my infant child taught me: All unhappiness comes from unmet expectations. I learned to set my mother free of my expectations. I set my father free of my expectations. I now have an incredibly close and loving relationship with my whole family because of setting all of us free from my expectations.

Integration Exercise: Evaluate Your Expectations

My story is not unusual. I know because I hear all sorts of unmet expectations in my office. I have patients who have bodies that are not meeting their expectations, who aren't getting the outcomes they expected for their efforts, are upset that insurance companies don't cover anything the way they expect, and so on.

Think about your personality type. Do you expect people to be cordial to you? Do you expect great customer service? Do you smile at or greet others with the expectation your smile and greeting will be returned in kind? Do you expect the stock market to behave in a certain way? Do you expect your husband to read your mind, your kids to behave, and the educational system to operate as you would like it to? Do you have expectations of your local and federal government? Of people, of organizations, of churches? If you are kind to others, do you expect others to be kind to you?

How often do you find your expectations are not met? How often are you triggered by an unmet expectation? Is it true that people are here to behave in the ways you expect them to? The answer is no. You only have control over your own behavior. That's it. You do have choices about what to do if your expectations are not met. You can change your expectation, or you can leave the situation you are struggling with. Just remember, wherever you go, there you are. Choosing to shift your expectations is the growth opportunity. Choosing a different environment comes with the high risk that you will find the same situations repeated. Why? Because you are there, and didn't learn anything the last time.

Use your journal and spend some time going through events, situations, and people in your life that didn't meet your expectations. If you do this correctly, there will be days and days of writing. Now look for common themes. Find the beliefs that are behind your expectations. For example, I used to get very miffed when I hiked and hailed my fellow hikers with a hearty greeting and happy smile and got no acknowledgment back from them. I used to mutter sarcastically under my breath. Why did I think that other people in the mountains would want to respond to me? Maybe they went into the mountains to get away from people like me, people who were needy for emotional connection. Maybe the person I just greeted with my Pollyanna good cheer thought I was too intense for so early in the morning. Maybe the person I greeted had just lost a loved one, a job, had just been diagnosed with an autoimmune disease or cancer. My need for a return of my greeting was self-centered. The greeting was not rooted in compassion and generosity if I expected something back.

Now when I greet someone with a smile, I have zero expectations of them. I am okay and they are okay, regardless of their response. Just remember that. No matter what, you are okay and so are the other people we share life with, even if it seems like they are not. They are on their path, learning their lessons. They are okay.

Take a look at the expectations you wrote and see if any of them can be shifted in the way I just described. Here's my guarantee: the more expectations you rid yourself of, the happier you will be.

Giving up Judgement

Judging and comparing yourself to others is so engrained that you may not know how often you do it. Pay attention to your thoughts. How many of them are a form of judgement? Do you see others as inferior to you in any way? Superior to you? More or less intelligent than you? Richer or poorer? Fatter or thinner? Older or younger? Do you judge the political or religious views of others as inferior or stupid? This list of examples of judgement just scratches the surface. Countless are the forms of judgement. Let's face it, there are subtle judgements happening under the surface all the time.

Why do we judge? Because we are trying to control our environment, make sense of it to achieve a sense of safety. We also judge because we are afraid of *being* judged. Fear of being judged causes a great deal of suffering. If you are afraid another person, or God, will judge you harshly, it causes disease within. I have witnessed in my life, in my clinical practice, and in spiritual communities I have belonged to that those who are most afraid of being judged are the ones who judge others most harshly. When you are unified with spirit, there is a complete absence of judgement. Judgement is strictly a function of the mind, of the ego. Learning to release the venom that arises from within, that causes you to judge yourself or another, is well worth the effort. The reward is brilliant, radiant, loving energy and light, more precious than diamonds, more precious even than the Kashmir diamond.

SECTION IV:
Solving the Puzzle
by Healing Your Hurt

"Healing takes courage, and we all have courage, even if we have to dig a little to find it."

~TORI AMOS

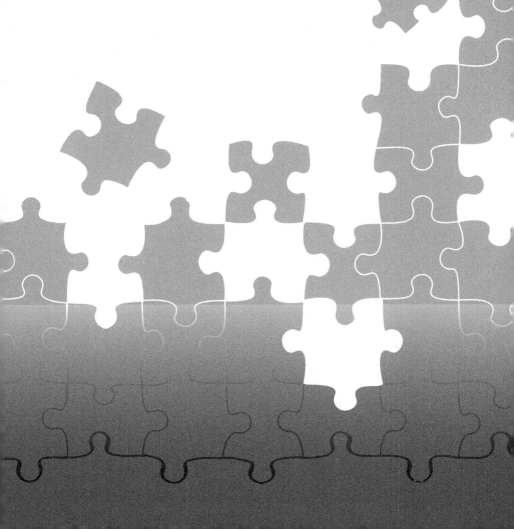

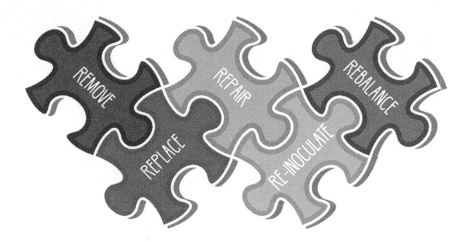

You have now framed your puzzle. You have the corner pieces in place. You are filling in the center pieces by fitting them into the framework. You are working on a strong foundation that holds your puzzle stable where you can observe it as you work. Next, we will apply the 5 R's of healing to release the rigidity of your mental and emotional hurts from your body.

As a reminder, the 5 R's are 1) **R**emove, 2) **R**eplace, 3) **R**epair, 4) **R**e-inoculate, and 5) **R**ebalance. Each of the next five steps in this chapter represent one of the 5 R's. You are putting them to work now.

In the last chapter, when I asked you to feel your emotions in your body, were you able to find where your body stores your experiences? Were you able to identify how old you feel when you are triggered? Some people struggle with this exercise. Why? Because as kids they learned to leave their bodies. It's much easier to live through stress if you don't have to feel it. You might be one of the people who are so adept at this that all feelings are experienced as thoughts, so you can stay in your head. You might just experience life only from your mind. If this is the case, the body and heart do not have a clear communication channel inside of you.

I often find women so dissociated from their bodies that all they can feel is pain. These are women who want to think their way out of every situation. But remember, the mind is what created the traps you are stuck in. You cannot expect the mind to come up with a solution to the puzzle it created. You need your *whole* self to do that.

If you were unable to connect with your body, don't worry. Just continue doing the exercises and be willing to self-confront. I will teach you an incredible way of using your past hurt as a mirror to help you free yourself of any pain you experience. I am going to teach you an elegant forgiveness tool that will help you release your body from dis-ease. It will also soften the hard defenses you have built over the years, which keep you from connecting to your heart and body. We are going to use the 5 R's of healing to create what you want to see in your puzzle, rather than what you have been creating as a default from your childhood mind.

CHAPTER 11

First Step of Healing–Resourcing

"If you can react the same way to winning and losing, that's a big accomplishment. That quality is important because it stays with you the rest of your life."

~CHRIS EVERT

Creating Mind, Heart, Body, Spirit Collaboration: A Step-by-Step Plan

Every woman is different. We each have our own hurts, our own beliefs that we made up about those hurts, our own ways of coping, and our own story of pain. The purpose of healing hurt is to free you from autoimmune disease. It's to soften the immune response system by turning down the sensitivity of the 4F stress response system. Have you ever been in a home with a sensitive smoke alarm? No one likes it when the alarm trips too easily. The following program will help you to turn down yours. The objective? To simultaneously turn down your immune sensitivity, to reduce the cortisol output that harms your gut lining, and to harness the power of epigenetics to alter the way you are expressing your DNA. And as a side benefit, to free you up from your trauma, so you can live a life filled with passion and joy.

In this chapter and the following four, we will apply the 5 R's of functional medicine to solve the missing piece of the autoimmune puzzle: healing your HURT.

Remove

1) Remove, 2) Replace, 3) Repair, 4) Re-inoculate, and 5) Rebalance

The first of the 5 R's is Remove. To remove childhood patterns of fear and resistance to life, you'll need to create a resource for yourself. This is essential. A resource is support or aid that can be readily drawn upon when needed.

You have doubtless experienced times in your life when you wanted more money, food, help, or emotional support than you could provide for yourself. When you are healing past hurt, you might find yourself in a position of wishing you had more support, stability, or calm within you. This next exercise is to help you build in that support. It's the calm place you will always carry within you, much like the calm in the eye of a hurricane. No one can remove it once you have created it. It's yours and it's forever.

Integration Exercise: Creating a Calm Space

As we begin to explore ways of healing past hurts, I would like you to have what is commonly called a "resource space" in your mind, heart, and body that you can access if you feel your memories or emotions are too strong to handle. This space you will create is your own personal private space that you alone can access. No one else is permitted in this space unless you invite them in. It is here that you will be able to connect with your wise older self, your spiritual connection if you have one, your child self, or to self soothe if you are upset.

The Steps:

1. First visualize a relaxing, calm place. Some people choose a mountain top, some a beach, others a forested area next to a babbling brook, and still others a meadow where they can sit with their back against a big tree. This space is meant to be relaxing for you. Do not choose a place such as your house or anywhere you have lived with other people. Instead create a secret garden outside of your house that no one else has access to. Or build a house that is only yours and is suited for your unique needs. Your calm place can be a place in nature you have been to before or it can be a place from your imagination. You get to build it for yourself. It is for you and for you alone. Write about your ideal calming space here:

_____

_____

_____

_____

_____

_____

_____

_____

2. Once you have picked a place, begin to construct it in your imagination.
    Visualize it to the best of your ability. Use all five of your senses. What
    colors do you see? What sounds do you hear? What do you smell when
    you inhale the air of your private relaxation place? What does it feel
    like on your skin, in your hair, under your feet? Can you taste what it
    is like to be there? Take your time. Close your eyes and paint your own
    safe space.

    For example: One of my calm, safe places (you can have as many as
    you can imagine) is a sacred site in Peru called Machu Picchu. When I
    began constructing my calm place within myself, I brought in the peace
    that I feel when I was there once all by myself at dawn. I drew in the
    light and warmth of the sun, the feeling of the cool, smooth, crystalline
    stones beneath my bare feet. I felt the energy of the rock formation I
    was sitting on permeate every fiber of my being from cells to soul. I
    breathed that power into my past, my present, and my future selves. I
    listened to the quiet, punctuated by the sounds of birds and the breeze
    in the trees. I pictured the vibrant greens, blues, and greys with the red
    pom poms on the brown and white llamas. I visually ran my hands
    over the textures and took in the scents. I tasted the air on my tongue. I
    placed the "crystal condor city" within me. I can go there anytime, no
    matter where I am physically. It is a resource.

    Now write about or draw your calm space, complete with all of the
    colors, sounds, textures, temperatures, visuals, smells, and tastes here:

_____

_____

_____

_____

_____

_____

_____

_____

_____

3. Now that you have created a calm space for yourself, ask yourself what
    you feel. Do you feel free, safe, calm, relaxed, peaceful? These are words
    I have heard when I take patients through this exercise in my office.
    What do you feel in your space of your creation? Name it. Say it out
    loud 3 or 4 times. This is your cue word for bringing yourself back to
    this place whenever you desire calming, soothing, or grounding.

    For example: *I feel grounded and centered in my own power and connection to
    the Universe when I go to my Machu Picchu resource place. I use the word "calm" to
    get there.*

    *When I am in Kenya, I get the amazing opportunity to connect with a variety of
    wild animals that are native to Africa. One of the most amazing of these creatures
    is the elephant. When I want to feel grounded, I just visualize a place I have created
    for myself in Kenya with elephants and say the word "Ellie" to myself three times.
    It instantly brings me back to that steady, grounded, maternal, and communal energy
    that I am wanting to resource.*

    What do you feel in your space? What is your cue word? Write it here:

    _____

    _____

    _____

    _____

    _____

    _____

    _____

    _____

4. Next, identify where in your body you have the sense of being in your
    calm, safe place. Take your time. Say your cue word either silently or
    aloud. Rest and feel your breath as it enters your body. Notice as it exits

your body when you exhale. Keep noticing, not struggling, just bringing awareness to your body. Where do you feel the peace of the place you have created for yourself? Write about it here:

_____

_____

_____

_____

_____

_____

_____

_____

5. Once you have found where you feel this sense of relaxation and peace in your body, give it a color. What color can you link to the feeling you experience in your private, safe space? Write it here:

_____

_____

_____

_____

_____

_____

_____

_____

6. Now breathe that color in and feel that area in your body grow brighter. Just rest here, feeling the calm, the peace, and the freedom of having access to a place that is in your very cells and is all yours. Write about your experience of moving this feeling through your body as light and color:

_____

_____

_____

_____

_____

_____

_____

_____

_____

7. When you are ready, open your eyes. Practice going into your calm place daily by saying the cue word either silently or aloud and then dropping into the place in your body where you feel it. Write about how you feel:

_____

_____

_____

_____

_____

_____

_____

8. Find a picture or a symbol that will remind you of your calm place. If it's a beach, do you have a shell you can place where you spend a lot of time each day? Do you have several shells that you can place in multiple places where you hang out? Can you find a picture on the Internet that looks similar to your place and print it out? Can you draw it, paint it, color it? Finding a symbol will help concretize the feeling and experience of relaxed calm, so you can resource it any time you wish.

Sometimes, when people have been through a lot of "T" trauma in their lives, it's difficult to create a place that feels calm, let alone safe. If you are struggling to do this exercise, don't continue. Stop and use the resource guide at the end of this book to find a therapist who can help you release your trauma. If the first therapist is not a good fit for you, try another one. It can take a few tries to find a therapist who feels right, who offers a balance of insight, support, and holding your feet to the fire. You deserve to have a life that is not defined by your past experiences. Don't give up on yourself. If you struggled with creating a calm place, please read on and learn how to practice containment. It will be a useful exercise for you to use while you are looking for and seeing a therapist.

Containment

Containment refers to selectively filing images, thoughts, or feelings that make you feel unsafe. I teach containment to some of my clients as a tool to help them stay emotionally stable when they are not in my office. The material in this book might trigger strong emotions or feelings that feel too intense for you to manage on your own. You can practice containment to dial feelings back, put disturbing images away, and stop ruminating on thoughts that interfere with your daily life. You only put them away until you are in a therapist's office. There, you can work through them with a trained professional who can help you process them properly.

The purpose of containment is to create a healthy boundary with your memories, your thoughts, and your feelings. It's not to suppress or rid yourself of them. Your life experiences—all your life experiences, including past trauma—are a catalyst for your personal growth and the expansion of your consciousness. Learning to process these experiences is part of maturing into a wise woman, a wise adult, an elder who will be able to help others.

I have listed several containment strategies. This is not an exhaustive list. You might find a method I have not listed that works better for you. Let your imagination lead the way here.

1. **Use your journal** to write about troubling feelings, images, and thoughts. Return to the pages you have written in your therapist's office when it's time to process these experiences.

2. **Create a container.** This can be an imaginary container or a literal container that you can decorate and embellish to your heart's desire. You can put a lock on it. It's only for holding any triggering or distressing images, thoughts, and feelings. Don't store your loose change in it. You can use a Mason jar, a shoe box, a cigar box, a bucket, anything you can think of. When I first learned this exercise in my own therapy, I created an imaginary jeweled gold trinket box as my container. When I had been through a particularly big growth spurt in my processing of past trauma, images would come up at night in my sleep. I learned to

stick them in my box, turn the little key to lock it, and go back to sleep. I knew that I could take them out the next time I had an appointment with my therapist.

3. **Connect to your spiritual guide(s)** and ask them to be the guardian of your traumatic memories. Ask that your traumatic memories be held safely until such time that you are in the supportive space with your therapist.

4. **What are your ideas for containment?** Write them here:

_____

_____

_____

_____

_____

_____

_____

_____

_____

If you get stuck with these exercises, remember it might be time to find a good therapist. You can check out the Resources Section of this book for some guidance. If you would like to take a deeper dive into your emotional healing, then I recommend you sign up for the **You Un-Broken** online course. Again, to reclaim your emotional freedom, you can register for the program in the Resources Section of the book.

Mentally Detoxing

"The wound is the place where the Light enters you."

~RUMI

Replace

1) Remove, 2) Replace, 3) Repair, 4) Re-inoculate, and 5) Rebalance

The second of the 5 R's is Replace. I have led you through ways to physically detox; now you will mentally detox to replace old toxic patterns with more nourishing ones. Continuous exposure to toxic thoughts is just as damaging to your health as exposure to the mercury fillings in your teeth. You must get them removed. The great news is you can. You can clean out your mental cupboard and stock it with healthy thoughts and beliefs, much like you can do with your kitchen pantry.

Integration Exercise:
Clean Out the Mental Cupboard

An average person has 30,000 thoughts per day. Of those thoughts, 94% are recycled—you have thought them before. Fear activates more than 1,400 physical and chemical responses, and it triggers a response from more than 30 different hormones. The toxic byproducts of toxic thoughts make you sick. Being able to detox your mind, build new neural networks in your brain, and activate inner bonding with yourself can help you increase resilience, one of the skills needed to reverse autoimmune disease.

I have given homework to some of my patients to list 10 things they like about themselves, and they come back with less than four. I have asked couples who are seeing me for therapy to write down what drew them to their partner when they first began dating. More often than not, at least one of the partners can't recall what they used to see in the other. When women are asked to write down 10 things they love about their bodies, I hear from them how easy it is to find fault and how difficult it is to find something to love. The list of criticisms is endless. The list of appreciations is limited.

Having a strong inner critic might keep you motivated to improve, but it can also be one of the triggers that sets off your internal alarm system, sending your body into 4F stress response system survival mode. Why? Because that inner critic is the voice that continues to let you know that you are not good enough. It's the one that says you must perfect the task at hand to be worthy. It's the voice you heard in your childhood. Your inner child is still cringing when you put those toxic thoughts on continuous loop for constant listening. You can call those thoughts automatic negative thoughts, or ANTs, and believe me, they will spoil your picnic. ANTs are what derail your train of thought, making it difficult to remember who you really are and what you love about yourself and your life.

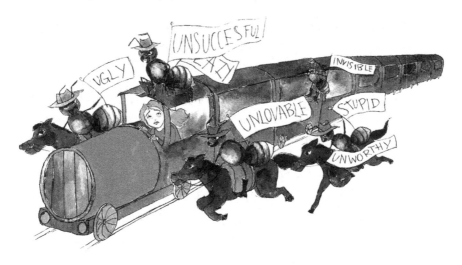

Detoxing toxic thought patterns and converting ANTs to automatic nourishing thoughts is just as important as detoxing toxic chemicals. A mental detox is not just about changing your thoughts. It's about learning to self-confront to pull out by the roots the habit of thought you created in childhood. When you are pulling weeds in the garden, you don't just get rid of what is above the ground. You pull the root up too, or the weed will grow back. Don't focus on just the behavior; get to the root by examining the motivation behind the thought. This will keep you from ruminating on the same toxic thoughts again and again. If you are recycling 94% of your thoughts, there is very little chance a new thought will attract your attention. Maybe this new thought is nothing great, but it may be a life changer. It's time to clean up the mind cupboard so you can see what's there, organize it, and throw out what is expired and outdated. That way you can fit new thoughts in there.

What's in the cupboard?

1. Have you made any "shoulda, coulda, woulda" statements in the last week?
   - "I should have _____."
   - "If only I had _____."
   - "I could have _____."

2. Have you thought any of the following (or any variations of the following) in the last week?
   - "I'm such a loser."
   - "I want someone else to take care of me."
   - "I need to play it safe."
   - "I'm unlovable."
   - "I'm not deserving of _____ (love, money, safety, friendships, God, etc.)."
   - "I'm not good enough."
   - "I'm too fat."
   - "I'm broken."
   - "I'm sick."
   - "I'm bad."
   - "He's bad" or "She's bad."
   - "At least I'm better than her/him."
   - "I have to be perfect."
   - "I am perfect."
   - "God loves me more than He/She loves ____."
   - "He/She deserves what he/she gets."
   - "I'm not safe."

- "Life is too hard."
- "Nothing ever goes my way."
- "Nobody understands me."
- "I have never had a happy moment in life."
- "Life isn't fair."
- "Why am I the only one who is suffering?"
- "If I am nice then others will be nice to me."
- "If I am fair then others will treat me fairly."
- "If my mother/father/husband/wife/sibling/child/God really loved me, she/he would know what I need."
- "I need to make everyone happy."
- "If I lose ___ pounds, or make ____ dollars, or get to vacation in ____, or buy this ____, I will be happy."
- "I know I'm right."
- "I'll start tomorrow."
- "It's all their fault."
- "I'll try."
- "Making a mistake will ruin my life."

3. Have you replayed a conversation or experience repeatedly in your mind? (Perhaps it didn't go the way you wanted it to, and you wished you had done it differently.)

4. Do you ruminate about past hurts?

5. In the last month, have you made a promise to yourself or someone else that you didn't keep?

6. Do you identify with an autoimmune disease, lack of memory, hormone imbalance, low level of energy, or an infection? For example: "my hot flashes," "my brain fog," "my arthritis."

7. In the last 24 hours, have you blamed something or someone outside of yourself for anything?

8. Do you feel like you have been victimized by life? Write about this.

9. Are you busy creating worst-case scenarios because you are worrying about something you cannot control in your future?

10. Is your mind passively letting time slip away?

11. Do you lack motivation and goals?

12. Do you believe you are inherently incapable of transforming your life?

If you answered yes to one or more of the above, it's time for a mental detox.

Here's the good news: you can change the direction of your train of thought by doing the simples exercises I am teaching you.

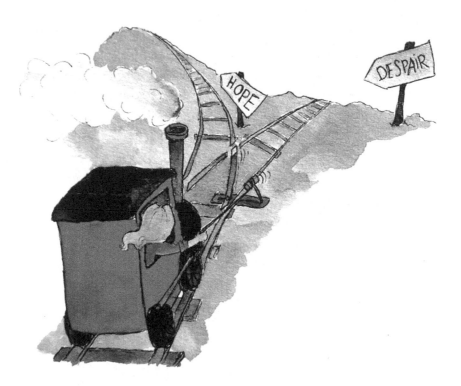

Using the 5 R's to Mentally Detox

Just as a reminder, the 5 R's are: 1) **R**emove, 2) **R**eplace, 3) **R**epair, 4) **R**e-inoculate, and 5) **R**ebalance

1. **Remove:** Look at the list of toxic thoughts above. Do you recognize any of them as your ANTs? If your habitual pattern is not listed, think of what thought patterns derail your train of thought. Write about them here:

_____

_____

_____

_____

_____

_____

_____

_____

_____

2. **Replace:** Rewrite your most common toxic thoughts to reflect a
healthy outlook on yourself and your life. Here are some examples:

- "I'm such a loser" gets rewritten as, *"I'm grateful for the opportunity I have to learn new lessons."*
- "I want someone else to take care of me" gets rewritten as, *"I am grateful that I can take care of myself."*
- "I need to play it safe" gets rewritten as, *"I am safe as I play with life full out."*
- "I'm unlovable" gets rewritten as, *"I am worthy and deserving of all of the love the world has to offer. I am infinitely loveable."*
- "I'm not deserving of _____ (love, money, safety, friendships, God, etc.)" gets rewritten as, *"I am worthy and deserving of all of the _____ the world has to offer."*
- "I'm not good enough" gets rewritten as, *"I am enough."*
- "I'm too fat" gets rewritten as, *"I love and appreciate this body that carries my spirit around and allows me to live my life."*
- "I'm broken" gets rewritten as, *"I am whole and complete just as I am."*
- "I'm sick" gets rewritten as, *"I am grateful for every breath I take as it means I am alive."*
- "I'm bad" gets rewritten as, *"I am a Divine creation, a child of God, and an angel on this earth."*

Now it's your turn. Spend some time replacing automatic toxic
thoughts with positive, gratitude-filled affirmations that create peace
and harmony in your nervous system.

_____

_____

_____

_____

_____

_____

_____

_____

_____

3. **Repair:** Now it's time to get to the root of your toxic thoughts. The meanings you made up in childhood led to the beliefs you have that contribute to your autoimmunity. Read through the Self-Limiting Beliefs column on the left of Table 4. These beliefs are only a small fraction of potential limiting self-beliefs or negative self-attributions. It is time to stop limiting yourself. You deserve to live the life you were meant to live. You have purpose here. It is your responsibility to share your gifts and to stop depriving us of your unique wisdom and greatness. It is time to awaken to your own brilliance and to let go of your expectation that others need to reflect your worth back to you. Self-worth is felt from the inside, not the outside. If anyone criticizes, condemns, or tears you down with words, and it affects your sense of deservingness and worth, you are listening to the wrong voice. This is the voice of the ego. Listen to what others say, search for the truth in it, and then leave the rest where it belongs—at their doorstep.

If you find yourself blooming like a flower when someone praises, compliments, or showers you with positive feedback, be careful. You will also wilt if you are criticized. Words have no bearing on your worth. You are lovable and worthwhile just by grace. You are a divine spark of God's essence. Only you can hide it under a barrel.

Repair any self-limiting beliefs that you resonate with in this chart by replacing them with positive ones. Repairing happens when you picture yourself as a small girl while you repeat the repaired beliefs. Speak directly to her. Repeat the positive beliefs at least once daily, out loud, looking at yourself in the mirror. Making eye contact with yourself in the mirror is important; see the little girl in the mirror through your eyes. If you have not been friends with the woman you see in your mirror, this is your opportunity to see your own divine essence and to repair any past patterns. Your eyes are said to be the mirror to your soul. Look deeply and encounter the light you are. This is a skill that must be practiced. Connect in this way with your inner goddess every day until it becomes comfortable and natural. Write your new beliefs here so you can practice them at least once daily in the mirror.

_____

_____

_____

_____

_____

_____

_____

_____

▼ **Table 4:** Swap your toxic, self-limiting beliefs with nourishing and life-affirming ones

SELF-LIMITING BELIEFS	POSITIVE BELIEFS
I cannot trust; people are not trustworthy.	I trust that all I experience is for my higher purpose, which I might not understand until later.
I am sick; my body, mind, or spirit are unwell.	My body is healthy, my mind is brilliant, my heart is open, and my soul is peaceful.
I am not safe; the world is not safe.	I feel safe and protected in the world. My positive thoughts ensure my well-being and the safety of my spirit.
I am alone; I am often abandoned.	I am connected always to those whom I love and to those who love me—and to the divine within me.
I am afraid my needs will not be met.	I feel gratitude for the Universe that meets my needs as I act for myself and release expectations for how things will transpire.
I am guarded; anything can go wrong.	By being vulnerable and going outside of my comfort zone, I am empowered.
I am pessimistic; if things can go wrong, they usually do.	Everything happening now is happening for my ultimate good and making me a wiser person.
I am a victim; people tend to hurt me.	I set healthy boundaries and release people that are toxic towards me from my life.
I am not enough; I never measure up.	I can do anything I set my mind to.
Life is not enough; I am dissatisfied.	I love and accept myself just as I am. I am grateful for life, just as it is.

SELF-LIMITING BELIEFS	POSITIVE BELIEFS
I will not forgive; I might get hurt again.	I forgive those who have harmed me in my past, and I peacefully detach from them.
I am angry; there is much to be angry about.	I am the architect of my life; I build its foundation and choose its contents.
I am overwhelmed; there is too much to do.	I am perfect as I am.
I am bitter; I have often been betrayed.	My ability to conquer my challenges is limitless.
I am resentful because I work harder than others.	My potential to succeed is infinite.
I am entitled; I have had more than my share of hard times and now deserve what's rightfully mine.	Everything in my life, and life itself, is an infinite gift that can never be earned or repaid.
I am unworthy.	I am worthwhile just by grace.
I am not deserving; I am not good enough.	I deserve all the love and abundance available in the Universe just by grace.
I am not lovable.	I am completely lovable and fully fabulous!
I am not loving.	I am a radiant being of love and light.
I am powerless.	I am powerful and strong.
I have to be tough because it's eat or be eaten out there.	I speak my truth with love and compassion, always.
I am closed off; it's not safe to show myself.	I show my authentic self to others and trust that those who stay are the ones meant to be in my life.
Other:	Other:

4. **Re-inoculate:** When we are healing leaky gut, we talk about re-inoculating your gut with healthy bacteria. I am going to give you 10 mental habits that I call mind traps that you can give up and replace with habits born from your heart that you can use to re-inoculate your mind. This will keep your mind free of the chaotic chatter of old toxic belief patterns. You are not a victim of your circumstances. If you are a victim, it is of your own mind.

a. Give up thinking in terms of right and wrong.
What if there is no such thing as right and wrong? What if truth belongs to each of us in our own way of perceiving? I can hear you respond, "What about murder?" In some tribal cultures in ancient times, human sacrifice was agreed upon as acceptable by the members

of the community. Were they wrong? In our culture the answer is "yes." We have agreed on a set of laws that we vote to amend. If anyone breaks agreed-upon laws, they are supposed to suffer the consequences. It doesn't make them wrong; it makes them guilty of breaking the law. There is a saying, "Would you rather be happy or right?" Practice letting go of black-and-white, only-one-way-is-the-right-way thinking. Instead, realize there are many 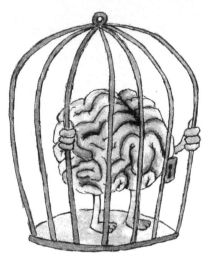 paths to the top of the mountain. Take your path and allow others to take theirs. Stand for what you believe in and live by your value system and let it end there.

b. Let go of the victim role.

Give up blaming: your health, your finances, your habits, your lack of education, and your feelings of insecurity or lack, events from your past, the opposite political party, the president, or God. You are the author of your own story. If you don't like how it's turning out, rewrite it. If you don't like your job, get a different job. But remember, wherever you go, there you are. The older you get, the more aware you will become that the same patterns repeat themselves, despite location changes. Why? Because you are present every time you are suffering.

c. Learn the art of radical acceptance.

The Serenity Prayer, written by Reinhold Niebuhr, goes like this: "God, grant me the serenity to accept the things I cannot change, courage to change the things I can, and wisdom to know the difference." This little prayer is a great one for people who resist what is. If you have a husband, like I do, who just cannot seem to put his coat away, you can be angry every single day about it. Or you can recognize that this is simply not going to change. And in the larger scheme of things, is it really that important? Is my husband here to teach me patience? Yes. I can then bow to him in my mind and thank him for being such an amazing teacher.

d. Notice your resistance to life and let it go.

Resistance to life shows up in people who are afraid of commitment. Relationship commitment issues such as divorce, frequent changes of employment, not committing to self-care routines, not being on time, finding fault in others, not finding "the one" romantic other are all examples of the exhausting pattern of resisting life. It's like standing in the river and trying to stop the flow; you can't. It shows up as ambivalence, such as an inability to make decisions, feeling stuck, frequent uncertainty, not knowing your own mind. It can also show up as overt resistance. You will find yourself saying things like, "I don't want to be here" in this _____ (marriage, job, state). When you feel that life is too hard, you are too exhausted, you are so overwhelmed, you are dealing with resistance to life.

e. The grass is not greener on the other side.

Appreciation for what you have and the life you lead is the surest way out of this toxic thought pattern. Appreciate your beautiful body. Appreciate your unique beauty and talents. Appreciate your abundance. Appreciate your opportunities, your friends, your lover, your children, your parents—for one day they might be gone. One of the most often repeated statements I hear from my elderly patients is, "I never appreciated my health or my youth when I was young."
When you compare, you despair. This means don't compare yourself to others who look like they have something better than you have. You never know what their story is. The irony is, it's likely someone is comparing themselves with you and wishing for something you have, creating suffering for themselves. Appreciate your life before it's gone.

f. Quit worrying about what others think of you.

What others think of you is none of your business. What you think of yourself is what is important. Seeking validation from anyone or anything outside of yourself will never work. For one thing, everyone else is running around seeking your approval and validation; how can they possibly stop long enough to fill your bucket? This sounds funny, but unfortunately, it's quite true. Everyone is busy projecting the image they want you and the rest of the world to see onto a screen and buying popcorn so you will not notice who they really are—just in case you won't accept them with their flaws.

It's very much like the Wizard of Oz. The Great and Powerful Wizard was just a little guy from Kansas pulling levers behind a curtain, keeping everyone petrified of his fake persona. Once Toto pulled aside the curtain and exposed him, Dorothy, the Straw Man, the Cowardly Lion, and the Tin Man all received lovely, folksy wisdom from him—answers they had each been seeking. Just live your authentic self and if someone doesn't like you, that's their prerogative. It has no bearing on your worth.

g. You cannot change other people.

The only person you can change is you. You cannot rescue people from their self-defeating behaviors. You cannot save them from their mental traps. You cannot motivate anyone except yourself. The truth is, when you are rescuing or saving another, not only will you fail, but you are doing it because of your own self-worth issues. This behavior keeps drama alive and well in your life.

Keep this in mind: Everyone has their own path to walk in this life. If you are constantly running interference so people won't fall, you are preventing them from getting to rock bottom. Often at rock bottom they will finally find the motivation they need to change. They are finally miserable enough and have destroyed enough that is lovely in their life that they cannot help but make the transformation you have prayed they would make all along. You need to offer help in ways that teaches them to fish, but don't bring them fish every day. Get out of the way. Focus on your own issues and work on transforming those.

h. Don't wait to be miserable before you are motivated to change.

Continuing from the last tip, make sure you don't have to hit rock bottom before YOU are motivated to transform the beliefs, behaviors, and habits blocking you from full self-realization, abundance, health, and love.

i. You are whole and complete, with or without a romantic partner.

If you are looking for your "other half" or "missing piece," you are destined for an unfulfilling life. Two strong pillars hold up the roof and stand on a strong foundation of relationship. If the two pillars are leaning in on each other, the roof will fall. You are your own soulmate at the beginning and at the end. In between you will have lots of relationships that will help you grow and learn about yourself. You are whole and complete.

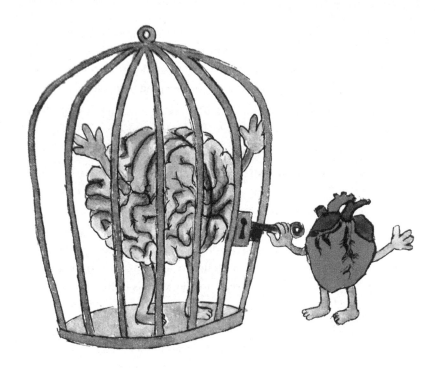

5. **Rebalance:** Each day rebalance your energy. You will come into contact with other people's toxic thought patterns and mind traps, from people who are not developing self-awareness the way you are. They will be at your place of work, in your home, or members of your community. Use the following exercises to clear your energy and clear your space. Choose just one and practice it daily; then check in to see if it balances you. If not, choose a different one. Keep playing with them until you find your own balance.

Tools for Clearing Toxic Energy

1. **Cancel, Clear, Delete** – Picture your mind having a keyboard. If someone says something to you that brings in toxic energy, hit the cancel, clear, delete buttons and wipe it from your screen.

2. **"Shields Up"** – Begin each day with an energy shield, just like in Star Trek. You are the captain of your own starship. Before you leave your home, ask your spiritual connection (Jesus, God, ascended masters, guides, angels, higher Self, Source) to surround you with a lovely purple amethyst crystal light. Amethyst is a crystal that has the energy

of protection. You can carry a small one in your pocket if you like. Any energy that is not loving will simply bounce off your shield and fall to the ground. Remember, you can make the inside of the bubble toxic with your own thoughts, so be aware of keeping them clear.

3. **Gratitude** – Shower all you see and think about with gratitude. If you are in a constant state of gratitude, it will shift any energy vibrating at a lower level.

4. **Motivations and Intentions** – Make sure you check in with your motivation for thoughts, words, and actions. Are you being kind to someone because you really want to be kind, no strings attached? Or do you expect something from this person? If you have any expectations, your deed is not motivated by kindness, but by desire for something. Set an intention at the beginning of your day to act as an instrument in the hands of God. Allow the Universe to play you, as Rumi says. Then your motives will be clear.

5. **Listen** – Make sure you listen for what is behind what others say. Their words may seem toxic, but what is motivating them? Are they afraid? Are they behaving in an unskillful way? Is there a way you can alleviate their fear and keep yourself grounded at the same time? Go for the win-win by really listening to yourself and the other. Can you recognize yourself and God in them?

6. **Breathe** – Breathing into the places that are tight, contracted, afraid in your body will help you to remain in your body when you are confronted with toxic energy. Stay connected and breathe in life-giving oxygen and breathe out your fear. If you keep your breath steady and deep, you can keep yourself from triggering your 4F stress response system.

7. **Love** – Keep the flame inside of your heart center burning. It's where you connect with God. Focus on that inner light and allow it to shine out to others. It is impossible to feel fear and love at the same time. Try it. You can't. Fear contracts you; love expands you. You can feel the difference in your body.

8. **Get Outside** – Going into nature and connecting with the elements, the earth, and the cosmos above transmutes toxic energy into beauty. The earth can take all our sh*t and call it fertilizer. The most amazing fruits and vegetables will sprout from it. Go outside, take off your shoes, plant your bare feet on the ground, open your arms wide, turn your

face to the sky, and feel the wind blow, carrying away your worries. Then lean over, place your hands on your knees, and simulate vomiting any toxic energy you have into the earth. Do this with gusto and even yell or scream it out. She will take it with gratitude, for she needs it to make flowers. Go into a body of water, or picture a body of water, and cleanse yourself of the toxicity. Then listen carefully for what nature has to tell you.

9. **Smudge** – Use a bundle of sage, incense, or a bell or singing bowl and walk through your environment clearing the energy out. Throw open the windows, place fresh flowers in the rooms, light candles, put on sacred music. Sit in meditation, prayer, and contemplation. All are wonderful ways of clearing out stagnant or toxic energy.

10. **Surround Yourself in a Crystal** – Before you go to sleep do a simple 3-part forgiveness exercise. First forgive others who have hurt you that day. Second, forgive yourself for taking on the hurt in the first place. And third, ask for forgiveness for any hurt you have meted out during the day. Then surround yourself in a crystal in your mind, set an intention that you will remember your dreams the next morning, and go to sleep with the intention that your amazing body will detox in the night and awaken refreshed and energized.

Write about the mind trips you encounter within yourself and from other people. How do they impact your life? What are the strategies that you will use to repair the toxicity you feel from within and from without? What are the loving strategies that you can access from your heart that will set your mind free of its life-long traps?

_____

_____

_____

_____

_____

_____

_____

Where you are today is because of what you thought yesterday. Where will you be tomorrow?

Reflecting

"What we see is what we have been looking for."

Repair

1) Remove, 2) Replace, 3) Repair, 4) Re-inoculate, and 5) Rebalance

The third R in the 5 R's is Repair. In this step, you repair what you perceive from others' actions. One of the tools for solving your autoimmune puzzle is the Mirror Exercise. You might have noticed it under the adaptive memory processing area of the HURT model diagram in Chapter 4. Mirrors are great for seeing our reflections. In preparation for the Mirror Exercise, let's start with learning to reflect. Taking the time to reflect allows you to see your own shadow. It illuminates where you are judgmental. Remember, judgment will show up as superiority and inferiority as you compare yourself to other people. This is a huge barrier to healing past trauma.

The truth is, every human being has the exact same personality traits. It's true. We are all mean, loving, cruel, joyful, happy, selfish, compassionate, stingy, generous, greedy, forgiving, and more.

There is a Cherokee tale that illustrates this point. It goes something like this:

One day, a young boy went to his grandfather and asked him how he could become a "good man" rather than a "bad man."

The wise elder said to his grandson, "My son, there is a battle between two wolves inside us all. One wolf is a dark wolf. It is jealousy, arrogance, greed, envy, resentment, superiority, inferiority, self-pity, deceit, false pride, and rage. The other is a white wolf: peace, humility, kindness, empathy, generosity, compassion, truth, joy, benevolence, and love."

As he watched his grandson absorbing this information, he added, "Whichever wolf you feed the most will be the strongest."

We all have the same personality traits; we just manifest them differently. When you are triggered about something another person has done to you, you might feel hurt or angry and say something like, "I would never behave in this manner!" When you find yourself thinking this thought, STOP! You have just begun to judge yourself as superior. Immediately begin to do this exercise and you will get under the real source of your anger, which is the softer and more vulnerable feeling of hurt or sadness. By judging in anger, you are trying to reclaim power in a dysfunctional way.

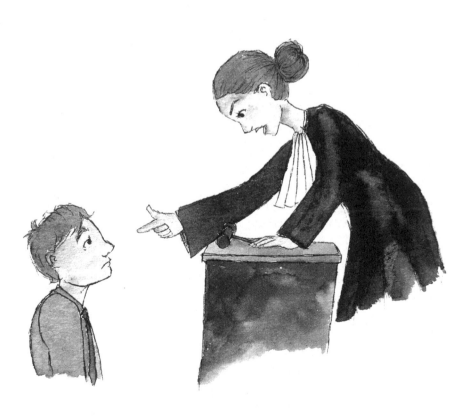

The personality trait of the "other" is demonstrated in a type of behavior that annoyed or hurt you. Likely, you will not do this precise behavior yourself and therefore can think you are not like the person who hurt you. However, go underneath the behavior and find what I call the ego or personality trait that drove the person to act in the way they did.

Example:

Let's use my sexual abuse experience that is part of my own story. If I picture my abuser and search for the personality traits that drove him to sexually molest me, I would list:

1. Uncaring
2. Weak
3. Unprincipled
4. Cruel

Now, if I use him as a mirror to *reflect* these traits back to me, I can search in my own life to see where these same characteristics show up. I do not look for the behavior; I look instead for the trait that *motivated* the behavior. For example, I have not sexually molested anyone and therefore not carried out that *behavior*. However, I have been uncaring, weak, unprincipled, and cruel in my life, just as every human has. Let's start with uncaring. When I am hurt, I can say things that are uncaring for sure. I have been weak. I have set exercise schedules for myself and broken them multiple times. I have made promises and broken them. This is both weak and unprincipled. I have been cruel in my life as well. In fact, I can remember being cruel to my oldest son when he was young and did something mean to our dog. I recall being furious and saying things I wish I had not said.

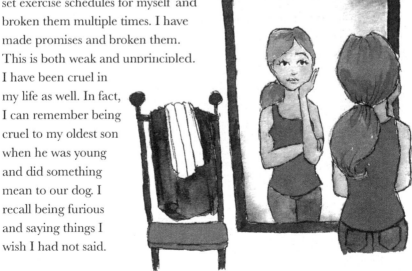

When you do this exercise, it is a great equalizer. When you have been hurt by another, it is quite easy to fall into moral superiority and hold them in a place of unrelenting shame and blame. This only hurts you, and over time, turns into toxicity in your body.

One of my favorite quotes is reportedly from Gautama Buddha: *Holding onto anger is like you drinking poison and expecting the other person to die.*

Seeing *yourself* as "the other" is an important step to real freedom from disease. Try these steps and use a journal to write about your experience. I recommend you start with someone who you are only mildly annoyed with. When learning to ride a unicycle, it is easiest to start with a tricycle. Start easy with someone not too close to you. The emotional upset will be less, and the exercise will be easier to process, if it's someone who isn't close to you. Starting with your mother, father, sister, brother, children, spouse, or other close loved one is a lot more difficult.

Integration Exercise: Reflection Exercise

1. What has triggered you? What behavior in the "other" has made you angry?
2. Think deeply about what would drive this person to do this behavior that you are offended, hurt, or otherwise upset about.
3. Identify that motivation in the other as a personality or ego trait. You can look at Table 5 for a variety of ego or personality traits.
4. Now take a few moments and see if you can find that same personality trait in yourself. Your behaviors will be quite different, so don't confuse behavior for trait. Again, focus on personality trait.
5. Write here about your reflections:

_____

_____

_____

_____

_____

_____

_____

_____

_____

I will give you the complete Mirror Exercise after you have completed some reflection. One step at a time; there is no rush. Take your time and really integrate this and the previous sections before moving on. When you are ready, we will begin working on a deeper level, self-confrontation and forgiveness, with the goal of helping you reverse the inflammation in your body as you eliminate the inflammation in your mind.

Once you have learned to reflect, you won't be trying to communicate from the 4F Stress Response System, or from the mind of an upset child. You will be more equipped to have an authentic conversation about what upset you from an adult place of sticking to your feelings and not blaming and shaming others around you.

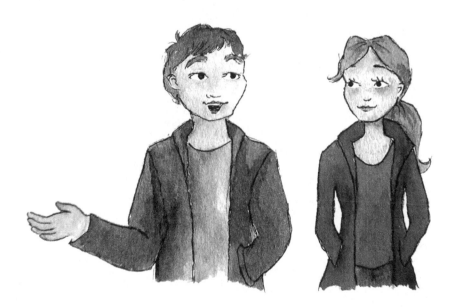

▼ Table 5: Negative Traits

Abrasive	Dogmatic	Malicious	Sanctimonious
Abrupt	Domineering	Mawkish	Scheming
Abusive	Dull	Mealy-mouthed	Scornful
Aggressive	Easily Discouraged	Mechanical	Secretive
Aimless	Egocentric	Meddlesome	Sedentary
Aloof	Envious	Melancholic	Selfish
Amoral	Erratic	Messy	Self-indulgent
Angry	Escapist	Miserable	Shallow
Anxious	Excitable	Miserly	Shortsighted
Apathetic	Extravagant	Misguided	Shy
Arbitrary	Extreme	Mistaken	Silly
Argumentative	Faithless	Money-minded	Single-minded
Arrogant	False	Monstrous	Sloppy
Artificial	Fanatical	Moody	Slow
Asocial	Fanciful	Morbid	Sly
Blunt	Fatalistic	Muddle-headed	Small-thinking
Bullying	Fawning	Naive	Steely
Brittle	Fearful	Narcissistic	Stiff
Calculating	Fickle	Narrow-minded	Strong-willed
Callous	Fiery	Negative	Stupid
Cantakerous	Flamboyant	Neglectful	Submissive
Careless	Foolish	Neurotic	Superficial
Childish	Fraudulent	Nihilistic	Suspicious
Cold	Frightening	Obnoxious	Tactless
Colorless	Frivolous	Obsessive	Tasteless
Complaining	Gloomy	Obstinate	Tense
Compulsive	Graceless	Odd	Thoughtless
Conceited	Grand	One-dimensional	Timid
Contemptible	Greedy	One-sided	Treacherous
Conventional	Grim	Opinionated	Troublesome
Cowardly	Gullible	Opportunistic	Unappreciative
Crafty	Hateful	Oppressive	Uncaring
Crass	Haughty	Over-imaginative	Uncharitable
Crazy	Hedonistic	Paranoid	Unconvincing
Critical	Hesitant	Passive	Uncooperative
Crude	Hostile	Pedantic	Uncreative
Cruel	Ignorant	Perverse	Unctuous
Cynical	Imitative	Petty	Undisciplined
Decadent	Impatient	Plodding	Unfriendly
Deceitful	Impractical	Pompous	Ungrateful
Demanding	Imprudent	Possessive	Unhealthy
Dependent	Impulsive	Power-hungry	Unimaginative
Desperate	Inconsiderate	Predatory	Unimpressive
Destructive	Incurious	Prejudiced	Unlovable
Devious	Indecisive	Presumptuous	Unmannered
Difficult	Indulgent	Pretentious	Unprincipled
Disconcerting	Inert	Procrastinating	Unrealistic
Discontented	Inhibited	Profligate	Unreflective
Discouraging	Insecure	Provocative	Unreliable
Discourteous	Insensitive	Pugnacious	Unrestrained
Dishonest	Insincere	Puritanical	Unstable
Disloyal	Insulting	Quirky	Vacuous
Disobedient	Intolerant	Reactive	Vague
Disorganized	Irascible	Regimental	Venomous
Disrespectful	Irrational	Repressed	Vindictive
Disruptive	Irresponsible	Resentful	Weak
Dissonant	Irritable	Ridiculous	
Distractible	Lazy	Rigid	
Disturbing	Libidinous	Sadistic	

The Mirror Exercise

"Adversity is resistance training in your
spiritual gymnasium."

Re-inoculate

1) Remove, 2) Replace, 3) Repair, 4) Re-inoculate, and 5) Rebalance

The fourth R of the 5 R's of healing is Re-inoculate. In this step, you will take the work you did in step 3, learning to reflect and repair your perceptions, a bit deeper. You will re-inoculate your mind with new ways of understanding yourself so you can move easily into the rebalance step.

We're All Human

Being human means we will have adversity, conflict, and suffering in our lives. It's part of life on planet earth. I often see my patients suffering more than they need to because they judge the stress in their lives as "bad." Actually, as I mentioned in Chapter 2, stress is necessary to strengthen your body, mind, and heart. Why do we need cardiovascular exercise? To strengthen our cardiovascular system, or heart. Why do we need weight, or resistance, training? To grow muscle and protect ourselves from bone loss. Well conflict with other people is your spiritual gymnasium. Adversity is God sending your spirit to the gym to expand your consciousness and strengthen your spirit. Learning how to interact with your shadow, and even to embrace and love it, builds spiritual stamina and resilience, which translates to a body that is healthier.

Let's return to the concept that all humans have the same personality traits that we manifest in different ways from one another. An example of this that is easy to understand is to take a figure in history who spent a great deal of time feeding his dark wolf, a figure that most can agree had some less than admirable personality or ego traits, Adolf Hitler. While Hitler might have had some loving qualities, these are not the ones that history has remembered. I use Hitler as an example because there has been irrefutable proof of his crimes against humanity documented with horrifying detail.

If you were to pull Hitler up in your mind's eye, what are the first traits you come up with that would describe his ego? When I do this with a patient, I discourage them from characterizations like "evil." What I am asking you to do is to really focus on his ego characteristics rather than his behaviors. In other words, what is it in his personality that would drive him to commit the crimes he committed against his fellow human beings? Why did he feel his criminal behavior was justified?

Some of the personality traits I came up with the first time I did this exercise were, "misuse of power," "cruel," "racist or bigoted," "angry," "manipulative," and so on.

If we all have the same ego traits that are manifested differently, then the next step is to look at this person as if they are a reflection or a mirror of yourself. As I look at Hitler with the recognition of some parts of his personality, I am looking for those same traits within myself. What makes this difficult for many people is looking beyond the behavior all the way to the ego or to the root cause of the behavior. When I take a hard look in my internal mirror, can I identify in myself those same characteristics I saw in Hitler? Absolutely!

For instance, the first time I did this exercise, I found an instance of mis-using power that very morning. In an interaction with my oldest son, I had played a formidable guilt card: "I would like you to spend time with your family rather than your friends this Spring break because soon you will be gone to college and we won't be seeing much of you."

Parents misuse power every time their requests evoke guilt. You can just hear that dark wolf howling with pleasure. Upon this realization and before the echoes of the howling shaggy black wolf had died out, I dialed my son's cell phone and had a wonderful conversation with him. I apolo-gized for my misuse of power and called it what it was. I explained why I had come to this realization, and ended the conversation by inviting him to call me out on this behavior if he ever witnessed it again, so that we could both be free of it.

Hitler was a masterful teacher for me. I have spent many long hours of my life, starting in high school after reading "The Rise and Fall of the Third Reich," grieving for the needless loss of innocent life at his hands, getting angry over his cruelty, and being frustrated in my search for meaning in the parts of history he and others like him had starred in. I realized during this exercise that he was simply a mirror of me and all other humans. He and every other human on the planet, whether characterized as saintly or evil, were simply reflections of each of us. We are each other's teachers.

After this first part of the Mirror Exercise, I could see that Hitler was me. I could bow to him and thank him for this insight and even forgive him finally. This does not mean that I need to or ever will forgive his actions or strive to emulate him. I simply know that the characteristics he had I also have. By being almost a caricature of those traits, he brought into sharp relief what we as a human race disown about ourselves. He became a teacher who reached thousands. His acts against humanity brought humanity together in a common cause and forced us to look at ourselves collectively and go deep with self-inquiry. He failed so miserably in what Joseph Campbell calls the hero's journey that he got our attention much too late in the game. We could not believe that the atrocities he was committing were true, despite escalating evidence that they were happening. His shadow was so long and dark that people didn't even recognize it as a shadow. His projection was so strident that the people around him saw only what he projected and didn't question who was behind the curtain. This plays out on political stages repeatedly, current time included.

When I moved on to work with "cruelty," I could find this trait even more readily. I can be mean, and the more I am cornered into having to look at my own shadow, the meaner I can be. This was quite a realization for me. I had to sit with my behavior and look intently into the reflection provided to me by Hitler. While I have never killed another person, or bought tanks and invaded Poland, I have been cruel in my dealings with my fellow humans— sometimes intentionally and sometimes inadvertently. The Mirror Exercise was a profound awakening for me to take full responsibility for my behavior and my own cruelty and to stop projecting it onto others. I had a long talk with my husband, who naturally bears the brunt of my bad moods. I invited him to also call me out if I stepped over the line that separates healthy conflict from cruel verbalization of frustration.

Looking into the mirror and seeing bigotry reflected back was difficult. I had always considered myself race neutral. I grew up in the military and had moved 21 times by the time I was 14 years old, including overseas and in the deep south. I had been on the receiving end of racism countless times by the time I was 14 years old and really thought I had learned how to navigate cultures without stepping on toes. A political election showed me the error in my ways right at the time I was learning to do this work.

The community I lived in was distraught about the outcome of a national election and I was treating many of my patients for depression. In fact, I coined a term for it: "post-electoral depression." When I looked at the reflection this election was revealing about my community, I knew in a flash of clarity that I was just as bigoted as the people I had voted against. By seeing them as different than I was, by polarizing, by embodying the same reactive energy I saw in them, I was fast becoming what I didn't like in them. In fact, I was them. I was bigoted against bigots, which made me a bigot.

This shocked me, and I saw once again the beauty in the reflection Hitler provided. Whatever energy I spent being angry with him was the same energy that made me him. The special place in my heart that had a wall around it, which contained the Hitlers of the world, broke open. It was no longer necessary to guard myself against anyone else's energy. If I just sent love and compassion in their direction, along with the knowledge that they are me, then I can be free of hate. (Why spend time hating myself?)

Behaviors I disagree with can be dealt with by having healthy boundaries. Instead of reacting in kind, I can spend my time in activities that enhance the human experience. I can gratefully bow to this long-dead fascist leader of Germany with appreciation for the lesson he gave me. I can feel forgiveness for the man and recognize the fortitude within myself that he inspired—to stand for unity rather than polarization. I can live my life as a statement of unity rather than from a place of polarization.

Working with anger and manipulation has become easier the more clearly I see my own shadow and reflection back from Hitler in the mirror. Anger is one of the human emotions. If you think of a symphony of emotions, anger might be the kettle drums and happiness the flutes. A symphony gets boring if there is only one type of instrument. Many of us meet anger in others with an escalated level of anger, in a misguided attempt to end their anger. A symphony gets intense if there are only kettle drums. The repression of anger into the body can be a trigger for autoimmunity. Learning to express your emotions in ways that do not make you sick and do not bring fear to others is a skill to be practiced.

I choose Hitler when I explain this exercise because he's easy to use. He's long dead. His victims are still healing and we as a collective consciousness can still feel the impact of his actions. However, he's several layers removed from day-to-day life for most of us. If this is not the case for you, please use another archetypal character who embodies easy-to-recognize shadow traits. There are plenty to choose from in the history of the world.

You will need to list every person in your life you can think of who you have had negative energy with. This will likely be a long list if you take time to reflect on it. Once you this start this process, events, people, and places will begin to emerge from your memory. You will be driving, preparing a meal, going about the tasks of your daily life and snippets will pop up. Write them down. The more you write, the more you will learn and be able to get to know the whole of you, both shadow and light. The more shadow you are willing to see, the more light you will be turning on in the dark closets of your psyche. The more lights you turn on, the more light will shine from you. You are becoming enlightened!

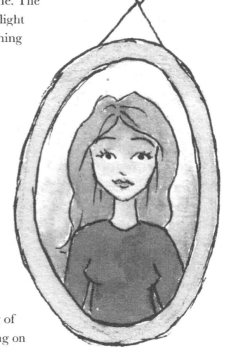

The need for a projector will disappear as you become the light people want to see. Remember that the brighter the light, the sharper the shadow. As you really get excited about getting to know the ego, it will become fearful as it feels its job security is threatened. Don't be alarmed. Go outside on a sunny day and watch your shadow on the sidewalk or the snow. Watch how it lengthens when the sun is lower on the horizon. This represents the beginning of your work. You have started turning on those lights in your shadow closets of your mind. However, when it is high noon, your shadow almost disappears. This is when you are no longer afraid of your shadow and have befriended and integrated it into your entire self.

> *"We tend to wear suits of armor, one over the other...*
> *We hope we will not have to completely undress."*
>
> ~CHOGRAM TRUNGPA

Integration Exercise: The Mirror Exercise

Remember that the personality trait of the "other" will have been demonstrated in a type of behavior that bugged, annoyed, or hurt you. You will likely not do this *behavior* yourself and therefore think you are not like this other person. However, go underneath the behavior and find the *trait* that drives the behavior. Therein lies the treasure of self-knowledge.

Here are the steps to the MIRROR Exercise (it is the Reflection Exercise from Chapter 14 taken deeper):

1. Identify the trait in the person you are upset with. Not the behavior; rather, the personality trait.
2. Write those traits down in your journal.
3. Note whether you see this trait in other people too.
4. Now look at yourself in the mirror of their heart. How do you manifest this same trait? This will also be called your dragon, demon, or shadow.
5. Now that you know how it feels to be on the receiving end of that trait, commit to watching for it in your life and to releasing it.
6. Now that you have seen yourself as equal to this person, is it easier to forgive him or her? You do not need to reconcile, but can you forgive?

Forgiving the "other" is NOT reconciling. You only reconcile if the person who has hurt you has apologized for the places he or she was out of integrity and established emotional and physical safety. If that has not been done, it is your responsibility to set healthy boundaries with this person and move on in your life. Forgiving is removing the toxic beliefs and feelings from your mind, heart, body and spirit so you do not get sick. Write about your experience with the Mirror Exercise here:

_____

_____

_____

_____

_____

_____

_____

_____

_____

_____

_____

You will learn the Freedom Forgiveness method in the next chapter.
Spend time here first. It is necessary before moving on to forgiveness work.

Congratulations autoimmune puzzle solvers! You have made it into
the center of your puzzle and yourself, where spirit dwells and your light
burns brightly.

*"God dwells in you, as you, and you don't have to 'do'
anything to be God-realized or Self-realized, it is
already your true and natural state. Just drop all seeking, turn your attention inward, and sacrifice your mind
to the One Self radiating in the Heart of your very
being. For this to be your own presently lived experience,
Self-Inquiry is the one direct and immediate way."*

~RAMANA MAHARSHI

CHAPTER 15

Connecting to All of Your Parts

"Repression is not the way to virtue. When people restrain themselves out of fear, their lives are by necessity diminished. Only through freely chosen discipline can life be enjoyed and still kept within the bounds of reason."

~MIHALY CSIKSZENTMIHALYI

Rebalance

1) Remove, 2) Replace, 3) Repair, 4) Re-inoculate, and 5) Rebalance

The final R in the 5 R's of healing is Rebalance. You are going to learn to rebalance your own equilibrium so that you do not rely so much on others to do it for you. This is true spiritual strength training.

Consider athletes who compete at the Olympic level, or musicians who perform at Carnegie Hall. How about actors who receive Academy awards or scientists and other thinkers who are awarded Nobel prizes. A great deal of practice and work has been put in before these awards are given. People do not *suddenly* become overnight successes. Likewise, a woman is never *suddenly* sick with an autoimmune disease. And it is equally unlikely that she will suddenly healed. It takes time to heal. It takes time to build new connections in the brain. It takes time to connect to the body if the connection was broken somewhere along the way. Athletes talk about being in the zone. Writers and artists get in the flow. Where is the zone? How do you live in what Mihaly Csikszentmihalyi has termed flow, or that focused mental state of creativity and happiness?

As innocent children, we live in a state of flow naturally. We don't have to seek for the zone because we are in it. It is through life experience, our interpretations of those childhood experiences, and the beliefs we create that we exile ourselves from a state of flow, from the zone of health, happiness, and creativity. To reclaim that state, you must learn to reframe your past hurts and reclaim your vital essence. This is done on a brain level, but also on a spirit level, by connecting to your source of the Divine that dwells within your heart. I am going to take you through an exercise that will help you to reclaim the parts of you that have been wounded and then to reframe your ACEs so you will be able to find the gift of what life has given you. Before I do so, I would like to address an interesting phenomenon: spiritual bypass.

Spiritual Bypass

I have a lot of spiritual patients in my community. They have been taught that negative thoughts bring negative outcomes. You might have learned that dwelling on hurt and pain will keep you hurting. You may already understand that forgiveness is vital for healing, but not have a full grasp of what forgiveness is and how to attain it. Many people remain stuck in their illnesses and inflammation, despite "doing everything right." Why? Because they are bypassing the pain, not processing it.

Spiritual bypass is giving lip service to spiritual precepts without actually detoxing the toxic beliefs from childhood. It's keeping your child self that experienced hurt in the past repressed. If you speak critically to your kid self when she pops up whining and judge yourself for having random negative thoughts or judgement, you won't be able to heal that leaky gut. People who struggle to heal do so because they are not starting at the beginning, they are hopping over the past and trying to begin with a clean slate. That works until your old childhood buttons are pushed, and then your 4F Stress Response System, which was wired long ago in childhood, is activated all over again.

By keeping one foot in the spirit world and one foot on the earth, you are in spiritual bypass. I speak of spiritual bypass as building a house on top of a toxic waste dumping ground. The building eventually gets permeated with toxic fumes because of the mess that lies beneath its foundation. You can also compare this to an abscessed tooth that has a crown placed on it. Eventually the infection will show itself and have to be cleaned out. You can get away with delaying the waste removal for some time, but eventually it will catch up with you. The Universe has a way of serving up the same challenge over and over again until you finally get the message that it's there for you to master before you can move on. Mastery of one level leads you to the next level of development. Your lessons become a bit harder as you master the lesser ones. This is because we do not stop growing in adolescence. Our minds and spirits continue to develop if you allow it. You can think of this like nesting Russian dolls, or Babushka dolls. When you begin to feel cramped in your current level of development, you will have a breakthrough that will propel you to the next size up. Eventually, if you are engaging in self-inquiry, you will begin to feel the pinch of tight quarters once again until you have a breakthrough. Physical illness is one of these growth catalysts. Usually, the Universe tries several gentler methods before dropping an anvil on your head to get your attention.

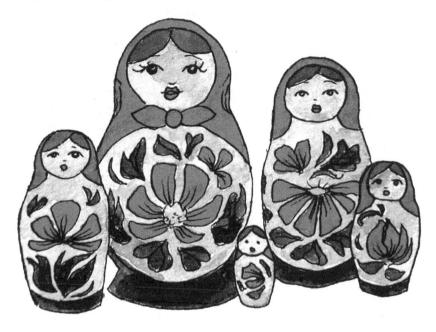

Your challenges are meant to help you grow, they are the weights in your spiritual gymnasium. There is a reason some people feel heavier to you than others. Do you remember your school days? Remember how you had teachers you loved, teachers you didn't really notice or remember, and teachers you vehemently disliked? Even though we didn't always love our teachers, they still taught us *something*. The same holds for the people we love and those we vehemently dislike today. They are all angels. They are part of the flower of life and have a place in the grid, just as you do.

The first step in this reclaiming and reframing process is to connect to your inner little girl. I resist using the word wounded child, because it's been used so much it is in danger of becoming a cliché. However, that is exactly who we are connecting to and healing here. But not just the part of you with emotional wounds; also the part of you who used to be in flow, who was innocent and knew she was amazing because the world was filled with wonder and she was curious to explore it. If your wounding goes back to pre-conception and conception, you will have to teach your little girl self how to be innocent, curious, and amazed at the wonder of life. You are learning to self-attune, or become the attuned caring and supportive adult in your life that you might still be seeking outside of yourself.

Integration Exercise: Self-Attuning and Connecting

If you typically have trouble visualizing, find old childhood photos of yourself and print an image from your computer that closely approximates your calming resource place. If you are visual, just follow along with the instructions of the exercise. Begin with the Confronting Your HURT Exercise you did in Chapter 10.

I asked you to go to a time when you had a distressing event in your life. You were asked to journal your age when it occurred and how you felt when you experienced the event. You were also asked to identify not only the emotion you felt, but where you felt it in your body. In Chapter 12, I asked you to create a resource place for yourself. You were asked to identify what you feel when you are there and where you feel it in your body. Your body is the record keeper of your life experiences. You are going to be using the information from these previous exercises to connect to your inner child, your older, wiser self, and your spiritual connection.

Connecting to Your Inner child

1. Begin with the child from the Confronting Your Hurt Exercise from Chapter 10. How old were you when this event occurred? What did you look like? What color was your hair? How was it styled? What did you wear at that age? Where did you live? What school did you attend? See how much information you can recall about that time in your life. What was your general belief about yourself? About the world you were living in? About your family? Connect to this little girl. Feel her

feelings. Feel her joys, her frustrations, and her confusions. What made her happy? What made her proud? What were her goals? Write about this here:

_____

_____

_____

_____

_____

_____

_____

_____

2. Hold the image of this precious child in your mind's eye (or look at a photograph). Remember how much she wanted to be loved, seen, heard, and approved of. What were her strategies to attain these? What decisions did she make about how to behave? Feel compassion for her. Love her, see her, and listen to her. What did she most need from her caregivers?

_____

_____

_____

_____

_____

_____

_____

_____

3. Now go to the experience you wrote about, the one where she was distressed. Walk in as your adult self and take her in your arms or by the hand and remove her from the situation that was painful for her. Take her to your calm resource place. How does this feel to both of you?

_____

_____

_____

_____

_____

_____

_____

_____

_____

4. Cuddle with her, sit with her, be with her in whatever way she needs. Quietly lend her your strength, attuning to her needs. Allow her to look around at the place you have created for all aspects of yourself, including her. How do you both feel?

_____

_____

_____

_____

_____

_____

_____

5. Now tell her what she needed to know back then. Tell her the things she would have liked to have heard from an attuned adult, but didn't. Let her know just how precious she is, what a gift to this world she is, how smart, funny, and perfect she is—just the way she is. If your wounding was in-utero, be there to accept her as a newborn into this world. Wrap her up and welcome her to the world. Let her know just how excited you are to help her light up and shine her gifts in the perfect way she is meant to. How do you both feel?

_____

_____

_____

_____

_____

_____

_____

_____

_____

6. Feel the love for this little one in your heart center as a glowing ball of light. Breathe that light throughout your body as you hold her, talk to her, and attune to her. Connect to her through time and heal those moments that need healing. There will be many of these. Take your time. Be patient. You will want to do this every time you are triggered, and believe me, there will be plenty of opportunities. How do you both feel?

_____

_____

_____

_____

_____

_____

_____

_____

_____

7. If you cannot do this entire exercise, do not despair. Sometimes there is so much self-loathing that you cannot attune to the little being you once were. If that is the case, you can access your older and wiser self and a spiritual connection who can help you. In the WILD Program, I have recorded some guided meditations for doing this if you need even more assistance. And remember, not being able to do these exercises is a signal for you to find an attuned therapist who can help you gain a sense of value for yourself.

The tree of life is an ancient symbol used by cultures around the world in mythology, philosophy, biology and is shared by spiritual traditions as diverse as mystical Judaism, Gnosticism, Christianity, and the ancient Celts and Persians. I would like you to visualize _yourself_ as a tree of life. The trunk of the tree is your neck. The roots of your tree draw nourishment from your heart center. The branches of your tree are your mind, with your thoughts being the fruit your mind bears. Ask yourself if the fruit of your mind, or your thoughts, are bitter and unripe or sweet and nourishing. *Figures 23* and *24* indicate how different your fruit can be if you are not fully connected to yourself in your heart. The love and compassion that you feel for your little girl will be drawn up the trunk of your tree and into the branches of your mind and bear beautiful fruit. If your thoughts are full of shame and self-loathing, then put them back on your tree and spend some more time with your heart. A newly planted fruit tree does not bear a large crop of luscious, juicy and nourishing fruit in the first season when it is still a sapling. This takes time and patience. Keep your focus on your tree and continually feed it the love that it needs and you will harvest a beautiful crop of fruit one day.

▼ Figure 23

Unripe fruit on your tree of life

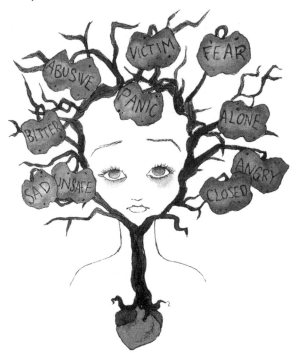

'The fruit of the mind that is bitter and
unripe ... think it over'

Ripe fruit on your tree of life

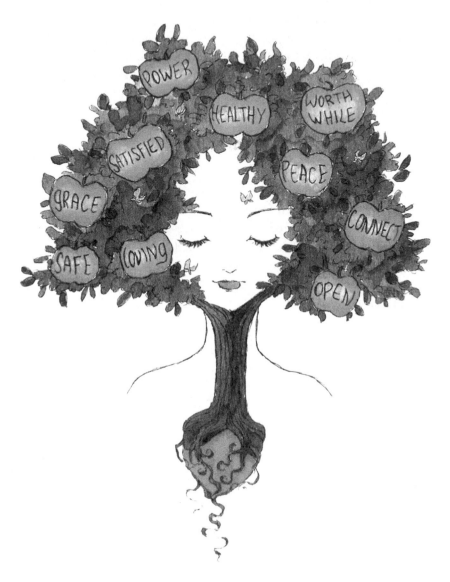

'The fruit of the mind that is sweet and ripe.'

Connecting to Your Older, Wiser self

1. I would like you to find an age that seems old to you. Now double it. You are creating a sense of what your essence is and this part of you is both ancient and timeless. This is your wise self. This part of you is the fourth layer of your pancha koshas. Have you ever met an elderly woman who has wisdom just beaming out of her? She did not get that in an instant. She lived a life that included self-confrontation and a willingness to learn from her mistakes and her hurts. This is where wisdom comes from.

   What age feels ancient to you? _____

   _____

2. Close your eyes and visualize what you imagine you will look like at 100 years of age. If you lived 150 years or 200 years what would you look like? Gaze into the eyes of this wise woman elder that you will become. What is remarkable about her eyes? What do you notice about her bearing? Her energy and presence? Her breathing pattern? Her smile? Her face? Her clothing and her hair? Her skin? Write all the details you can bring up about her.

   _____

   _____

   _____

   _____

   _____

   _____

   _____

   _____

3. Now ask her what she would like you to know. Just as you did for your little girl, you are now asking your wise self. What would she tell you about your present-day dramas and traumas from her perspective? What wisdom does she impart that you can use to connect to your little girl self? Bring them both to your calm resource place. How do you all feel?

_____

_____

_____

_____

_____

_____

_____

_____

_____

_____

4. Does your wise elder self have a gift for you? What is it? What does it symbolize? How are you to integrate it into your life? Thank her and show appreciation for the groundedness and perspective she offers you. Really connect to her. Create a time that you will meet regularly or ask her to send you a sign when she wants to speak with you. Turn to her whenever you are in need of a perspective free of ego and the impetuosity of youth. She is closer to heaven than you are; connect with her often!

Write about her gift, the symbolism of the gift, how you will integrate this gift into your life. When will you set aside time to connect to her?

_____

_____

_____

_____

_____

_____

_____

Connecting to Spirit

You may or may not have a sense of what a spiritual connection is. If you were raised in a religious household, you might still retain that childhood connection to the God or spirit of your youth. You might have rejected that

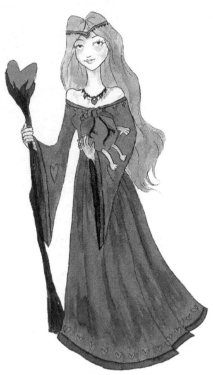

notion of God and created a connection that makes more sense to your adult life. You might have rejected spirit entirely in adulthood and have wounding or trauma that came from someone else's ideas of God. You may believe that your idea of God is the only correct one to follow, or you might be resentful of people who believe that their spiritual path is the "right one" and that all others are inferior, lacking the full truth.

None of this matters for this exercise. The only thing that matters is your awareness of your relationship to the final layer of your pancha koshas, your bliss sheath. This is the portal that connects you to the transcendent. Any toxicity in your body, energy, heart, and mind will keep you from having complete access to the kind of bliss that happens when you are one with God.

Now, this word, God, is a touchy one. I have used God, Universe, Divine, Source, Creation in my writings and teachings to try to make sure I do not ruffle feathers. However, if you are ruffled, this is your trigger and a source of pain that requires healing. Being willing to self-confront is key here. Making peace with God is often the unspoken theme of many of my therapy appointments with my patients. When I talk about God, I talk about the power that creates, that transcends time and space and earthly ideas of what is possible. I talk about the union of masculine and feminine, the radical acceptance that all IS God and that this infinite, boundless source of love within me is what I can enlist to learn from any pain, struggle, and trauma that I have had or will have in the future. So that I may become more and more a being that dwells in pure love and light.

When you were a child, experiencing distressing events in your life, you not only felt powerless, but you were powerless. It is the lot of a child to be under the control of those who are in authority and have learned how to navigate life, who are developmentally more advanced. This means you do not usually pick your own meal times, when you go to school, what you wear, what you watch, how you spend your time, when or if you brush your teeth and bathe, and so on. You are being taught how to live in the world and therefore, you are not the one in charge. As you grow, you will reach adolescence and begin to push for the autonomy necessary for that stage of development.

Attuned caregivers are aware of how to balance these developmental stages with love, listening, and compassionate boundary setting. However, no matter how attuned your caregivers were, they did not show up in exactly the way you needed them to 100% of the time. This is part of childhood. We spend our first 18 years taking on the wounds of childhood and the next 40 to 60 years learning what we are meant to learn from them. When you feel powerless as an adult, you are not your chronological age, you are back in those first 18 years of life somewhere.

Connecting to spirit is symbolic of connecting to something you feel is more powerful than you are. That's why your religion, spiritual path, or lack thereof does not matter here. You are learning to connect to a power source when you feel powerless. If you have connected to your little girl and to your older, wiser self, and are still coming up feeling short on power, then it's time to create or strengthen your connection to spirit. I am going to introduce you to Mark to give you an example of this.

Mark

A young man, who I will name Mark, came in to see me a number of times for anxiety related to his romantic relationship. As his story unfolded, it became clear that the meaning he had attached to what it meant to be loved was very different than the behaviors his partner was manifesting. Mark's beliefs and his partner's words, actions, and attitudes did not match. Knowing that meanings, beliefs, and behaviors are created in childhood, I asked Mark to tell me about how his sexuality unfolded when he was growing up.

He told me a story of the suffering he endured as a young boy. His tale gave me a glimpse of a young boy who was lonely and spoke often to the stars he saw as he gazed out his window at night. He knew he was different from the other boys at school and struggled to find ways to connect to them, knowing their energy levels were somehow mismatched.

As he began to mature, he realized his desire and attractions were different than the boys who were in the class room with him. He was attracted to boys in ways that did not just include playing baseball and riding bikes with them. As he gradually accepted his homosexuality, he felt ostracized by the children in his middle school. In class and on the playground, he felt left out and was bullied. He felt different from everyone else. When I asked him to go back to that playground to check in with his younger self, he felt sad about how lonely little Mark was.

I asked if he would like to provide little Mark with a spiritual connection to change the energy of fear and loneliness during that time of his life. He chose a black panther. He was delighted to give his younger self this powerful cat as a protector to take outside during recess time. He knew that no one would bully him again. And even better, he would not allow anyone to drain his own power. He could call on the big cat energy anytime he needed to from then on.

Mark came away from this session having provided a new sense of wisdom and safety to his inner, younger self. It allowed him to "cut the wires" to the button or trigger that had formed as a child when he didn't feel accepted or safe. As an adult, when he felt rejected, his reactions were overblown and scary to those around him. He was now able to calm his reactions and comfort the child part of himself that had experienced rejection. He changed his meanings and his belief about himself—and his behaviors, by enlisting the energy of a black panther.

My patients use their relationship with Jesus, ascended masters, angels, trees, the sun, Mother Earth, the elements, gurus, and like Mark, powerful animals. You can call on the energy of a super hero. You are using the archetype to instill yourself with the power you need to reclaim the perceived loss of power from your past, so you can then reframe your hurt into the gift that it can now be.

Use a journal to complete this exercise. I have recorded a guided meditation for doing this, and all of the other exercises in this book, in the WILD Program if you need more assistance.

1. Close your eyes and go to your calm resource place. Settle into the peace of your own private haven and heaven. How does this feel?

_____

_____

_____

_____

_____

_____

_____

_____

_____

_____

2. If you already have a strong spiritual connection, please invite that being to be with you. Who or what is this connection?

_____

_____

_____

_____

_____

_____

_____

_____

3. What is remarkable about this being or presence? What do you notice about your own energy in their presence? What do you notice about the feeling in your heart? Your mood? The rest of your body? Write all the details you can bring up about your spiritual connection.

_____

_____

_____

_____

_____

_____

_____

_____

_____

4. Now ask your spiritual connection what you need to know right now. Just as you did for your little girl, you are now asking from your spiritual connection. What would this being tell you about your current-day dramas and traumas from a spiritual perspective? What wisdom do you learn that you can use to connect to your little girl self? Bring them both to your calm resource place. How do you feel? What are the messages you receive?

_____

_____

_____

_____

_____

_____

_____

_____

5. Does your spiritual connection have a gift for you? What is it? What does it symbolize? How are you to integrate it into your life? Thank this being and show appreciation for the groundedness and perspective that you have been offered. Really connect, not from the need for spiritual bypass, but from a desire to self-confront and learn from your pain and hurt. Write about your experience and gift:

_____

_____

_____

_____

_____

_____

_____

_____

6. Create a time that you will meet regularly. Is this prayer? Is it reading sacred works? Is it meditation? You can ask for a sign for when you

need to reach out. Turn to your spiritual connection whenever you are in need of absolute unconditional love and acceptance. Again, your spiritual connection is closer to heaven than you are, connect often! And when I say heaven, I mean the state of flow attained within, here on earth. Write your intentions here:

_____

_____

_____

_____

_____

_____

_____

_____

_____

Well done! Next up, the secret sauce! Forgiveness is the final step in healing emotional wounds and reversing autoimmune disease, in fact any disease.

CHAPTER 16

Forgiveness–The Last Piece of the Puzzle

"Wholeness is not achieved by cutting off a portion of one's being, but by integration of the contraries."

~CARL JUNG

Forgiveness is a willingness to give up judgement, dissolve resentment, and release bitterness toward someone who has hurt you. Forgiveness is the ability to see the "other" as God and as one with yourself, thereby allowing yourself to ease into compassion, positive opinion, and even love.

Note that forgiveness is **not** about disregarding actions that have caused pain or forgetting that something painful happened. It does not mean excusing poor behavior or abuse. Neither is it reconciliation, which is not possible unless the perpetrator has taken responsibility for wrong-doing, properly apologized, and physical, emotional, and spiritual safety have been established.

People often resist the very idea of forgiveness because what they fear is reconciliation with someone who has demonstrated unsafe behaviors. Others will forgive through spiritual bypass, but fail to do the work to see themselves in the "other." Thus, they may wind up only building a crust over the top of the hurt and pain. You now know what happens when you do that; you get sick. The bitterness, resentment, and anger will eat you alive. This is why Confucius said, *"Before you embark on a journey of revenge, dig two graves."*

The process of forgiveness is one that builds strength and resilience. It shifts you out of the autoimmune mind-set. It is said that only the strong can forgive and only the weak seek revenge. The great Nelson Mandela knew that he had to forgive those that had imprisoned him and were imprisoning his people in apartheid. He said, *"As I walked out the door toward the gate that would lead to my freedom, I knew if I didn't leave my bitterness and hatred behind, I'd still be in prison."*

Mandela had learned that forgiveness was the secret sauce that would help him rewrite his story, help him reclaim and reframe his life from being a victim to being a leader. Real forgiveness, not lip-service forgiveness, allows you to find the gift in your suffering. This enables you to complete your hero's journey. Without real forgiveness, you will be doomed to continue circling the same maladaptive memory loop from the HURT model.

There are 3 kinds of forgiveness that must happen for healing to occur from the cell to the soul.

1. It is important that you forgive those who have hurt you.
2. It is essential that you ask for forgiveness from those whom you have hurt.
3. It is vital that you forgive yourself for taking on the hurt and keeping it.

Nothing in life is yours until you make it yours, including pain. It's time to get real about those childish meanings that were created a long time ago. It's time for beliefs that fit the adult you. It's time for you to create behaviors and habits that match your intentions and dreams for your life. If you are not living the reality you would like to be living, connect dots. Frame your puzzle, do the Mirror Exercise, engage with the Freedom Forgiveness Method at the end of this chapter, and identify every one of your self-limiting beliefs. Clean out the closet and throw out everything that you have outgrown, just like you are throwing out your autoimmunity. They are no longer yours. It's time to rewrite your story.

Rewriting Your Story

The last step of the Freedom Framework that frames your puzzle is to rewrite your story with intention, rather than from the perspective of an upset child. You have learned that the first step in authoring your own story with intention is to review the meanings you have made up about your experiences, the people in your life, and the world in which you live. Your story is of the greatest importance. It's the book of your life. If you are not satisfied with the way it's going, if you don't like the picture your puzzle is making, then rewrite it.

I get one of three responses when I work with people to discover meanings, beliefs, and behaviors that need to be rewritten. I have the "Teflon" client who had a "perfect childhood"; I have the "Velcro" client who attaches blame and doesn't want to release it; and I have the open and ready client who shows up with a journal and pen in his or her hand. Let's see which one you are.

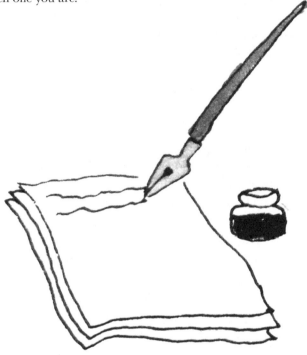

The Teflon Story Teller

As you have been reading this book, doubtless you have already uncovered some meanings that you created in childhood that you would like to recreate. If you do not, you might be having an experience like some of the people who have come to see me who say, "I had an idyllic childhood; there is nothing back there that is the problem." They will then follow up with, "the problem is my job, my spouse, or this disease I have."

By now you have probably seen that whatever you are triggered by in the present was set up as a "button" years before your job, wife, husband, or health issue were in the picture. Remember, you will emerge from even the most perfect childhood with meanings that are influencing beliefs and behaviors in your present life that no longer fit you. This is not about big trauma. It's about childhood interpretations of experiences through child brains that are not fully developed. Some of those beliefs might not fit your adult self. You are not blaming your parents. You are not betraying your heritage. You are not denying the incredible amount of support you might have received as you were growing up. You are just going through your closet and weeding out meanings that are outdated and don't fit.

If you have a hard time finding a meaning or belief too small for you, do the process from the other direction. Start with the "upset" you are experiencing in the present, and then reverse engineer it. Experience the current button that's upsetting you. When did you first have a similar feeling? What was that childhood experience? What belief did you formulate in your child mind at that time? What behavior pattern did you develop based on that belief? This is getting to the root of a pattern that is currently restricting your self-expression, balance, and health. If you have difficulty getting back to the root of this pattern, and you well might, because often it's buried in our subconscious, a good hypnotherapist can help. Please see the Resources at the end of this book.

This kind of mind that prefers to forget everything from the past is what I call the "Teflon mind." The direct opposite is the "Velcro mind."

The Velcro Story Teller

The Velcro story teller is someone that has a mind like Velcro. They hold onto the memories of their hurt and pain and have a hard time letting go, taking responsibility for their lives and forgiving past transgressions fully. I have a Velcro mind. It is wonderful for remembering what I learn, but not so great for forgetting what I don't need to hold onto any longer. The Velcro mind is great for learning tools for transformation. Use it when you need it, and then release the two sides of the Velcro periodically to clean out all of the debris, just as you have to clean your hair brush every once in a while. Let the beliefs and behaviors that keep you locked in your mind traps and on the lookout for danger be rewritten. Isn't it time to be free? Free to love, free to forgive, free to be friends with the woman you see in the mirror? If you are on the defense, it's hard to be friends with others or yourself. You are too busy looking for reasons to be offended.

The Willing Story Teller

We need *willingness* to get back to meanings we made in childhood. When a client who comes to see me sits down and says, "I have noticed this pattern getting in my way," I do an inward happy dance. This means I have an open and ready client. She or he inevitably has a journal and a pen and is ready to "get to work." Over time, this level of willingness leads to self-inquiry and self-discovery becoming play rather than work.

In the beginning, diving deep is a frightening prospect. We may worry we will be judged by the coach, therapist, or clinician in front of us. We may worry we won't be able to access anything "worthwhile" and make the whole session "a waste of time." Many of my clients worry they aren't "doing it right" and try to take care of me as their therapist and coach so I don't have a frustrating time working with them. Sometimes, it's not even conscious worry that stands in the way. We may simply have a subconscious fear reaction that keeps us from looking within and taking responsibility. This is often the case when a client was raised by a highly critical or abusive parent.

Naturally, the blocks holding you back from looking within will also show up in other areas of your life. When I am helping a client with trauma release, the best and most therapeutic thing I can say when a fear comes up is, "be aware of that (thought, belief, pattern, feeling, sensation, emotion, etc.)" Ultimately, the mind, heart, and spirit will come into coherence and communicate. The self-limiting patterns will unfold like a flower bud

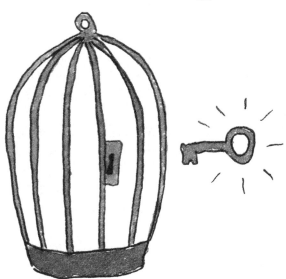

blooms. It will happen at the pace the mind is comfortable with. It is not to be rushed and not to be pushed away and ignored. Willingness means readiness to begin the process of becoming the author of your story in a way that matches your level of development. Willingness frees you from the cage of your body and your mind when you have autoimmune disease or any other chronic imbalance.

I would like to integrate the steps you have learned in this book. Let's walk through the process again, this time with Celia.

Celia

Celia was 30 years old when she came to see me with autoimmune eczema that had remained stubbornly resistant to every dermatological intervention she had tried. As with the other patients you have met, Celia's autoimmune puzzle also contained leaky gut, toxins, a genetic piece (mother also had eczema), and a history of trauma. Celia could be described as somewhat ready and willing to heal her trauma and reframe her story, but was still quite attached to holding onto her meanings and beliefs. She had not yet connected her behaviors to the suffering she was experiencing in her life. She had not recognized the pattern she was repeating, and was doomed to continue to repeat as long as she remained in Velcro mode.

Celia's parents were divorced when she was 10 years old. Her father moved away, and she lived full time with her mother and siblings. As an adult, she noticed she was often triggered when things didn't seem "fair" in her life. She might see how much money a co-worker was making and believe she should be making more because she worked harder. She compared what her siblings received from her parents and believed it was unfairly skewed against her. She saw more time, appreciation, money, and recognition bestowed on her siblings than came her way. One of her parents re-married, and as a result, she felt "unfairness" acutely. She developed an "entitlement" trigger that she didn't recognize, which went off like a time bomb without warning, keeping her feeling stressed, moody, unbalanced, and exhausted. She had autoimmune disease. Her skin flared with eczema when these episodes flared.

She had made up a meaning in her childhood. Whether she realized it or not, she had come to me to help her discover that meaning. Meanings will be written in your mind as "you are" statements or "life is" statements.

I started my inquiry by asking her how old she felt when she was triggered by this "unfairness" belief. She said she felt 10 years old. She recalled she was ten when her parents split up and made that connection.

I asked her to speak directly to the parent who she felt entitled to receive something from. In this case, she said it was her father, because her mother was left to "work hard and do everything."

I asked her to give her 10-year-old self a voice to express the meaning she had made up at that time. She said, *"Dad, when you left, I was glad, because you and mom fought all of the time. But you didn't give us enough support. You were not a good parent."*

From that meaning, I asked her to identify the belief she had created. *"My dad owes me,"* was her belief. This is a mind trap called entitlement. It was fed by both of her parents who tried to make up for the divorce by telling her how special she was. This fed her entitlement mind trap, because she made up a meaning that *"I am special and I am a victim of my dad's selfishness."*

Now there is a double whammy, because neither her mother nor her father helped her to see that she is no *more* special than every other person that lives on the earth. She is just that special. Her belief ultimately ends up as, *"My dad owes me because I am more special than any of the other kids and he has hurt me."*

The behavior Celia adapted as a result of this meaning and belief combination was to indirectly expect her father to be at her side when she wanted him, but she did not have to work at being there when she did not feel like it. She did not show up for holidays with him, didn't call on Father's Day, didn't get to know his family when he remarried, and worked very hard at maintaining her, "I am special and my daddy owes me" place in his life. She lashed out when anyone tried to point out the childishness of this belief and how it led to immature behavior in her adult life. Celia clung to the meaning, the belief, and the behavior, even at the risk of alienating her father and his family.

Our minds can wander down dark and treacherous roads that have been built by the engineer called the ego. I pointed out the mind trap she had caged herself in, and the obvious lack of freedom she suffered as a result. At first, she could not see it. She very much wanted to blame people and circumstances to justify her anger. I acknowledged her pain and her suffering and gave her space to feel it in her body, to feel what it was doing to her heart, and to recognize the fact that her own thoughts were destroying her peace.

Finally, she took on the challenge of rewriting the meaning she had created so long ago. She realized she had to give up the expectation of entitlement because it was keeping her trapped. She sat with the idea that her parents, future children, the world, God, her job, her body, her government, her significant other did not actually owe her anything. She owed herself everything. She was no longer a powerless child. It was up to her to take responsibility for her life and how she lived it.

"You owe *you* everything," I repeated softly. I had her adult self cradle her 10-year-old child self, telling her that she could now take responsibility for her life. She would be there for her when she needed it. She would provide, she would listen, she would love herself unconditionally as only she was capable of doing. She would meet her needs, be present; she would grow and expand her consciousness and break free of the victim trap she had been in.

She explained that the meaning the 10-year-old had made up was actually not true. It was just the best meaning she could come up with at the time. She lovingly and gently told her little girl self that dad and mom had not belonged together, and it had nothing to do with her. She did not need to be sneaky to get her needs met. She could just ask, take no for an answer, or accept any gift as an act of generosity, not a token of how much she was loved.

Her new meaning was rewritten as: *"I am able to ask for my needs in a healthy, articulate way. I give those around me the freedom to contribute to me and hold no expectations about what I receive. I know the Universe supports me abundantly and all my needs are already met before I even think them."*

Celia, having practiced living with this new meaning for a few months now, is poised to take my Integrative Medicine Health Coach Certification course. She wants to learn how to run the functional medicine labs she has done and benefited from herself. She wants to know how to make recommendations for others based on the feedback she is now trained to recognize in her own body, and based on the lab work she now knows how to read. She wants to help others transform their beliefs just as she has, so they too can find freedom from autoimmune disease. She is empowered and now feels the desire to empower others. She took a victimized, self-limiting meaning and rewrote it into a powerful one from which she built a powerful belief. She is now integrating what she has learned and is taking powerful action toward a purpose that vitalizes her.

Integration Exercise:
The Freedom Forgiveness Method

The following is the Freedom to Forgive Worksheet:

1. Tell your HURT story in as few words as possible. This is called the triggering event. Express your HURT aloud in one of the following ways:

    i. To the person who hurt you.

    ii. To an empty chair while visualizing the person who hurt you.

    iii. To a person filling in as a proxy for the one who hurt you.

    b. Keep it short and to the point:

    i. "When you (describe what the person did or said) _____

    _____

    _____

    _____."

2. Express the emotion you experienced or are experiencing now:

    a. "I felt _____."

    (make sure it's a feeling, not a belief)

3. The meaning I made up about this event is:

    "You are_____."

    a. The meaning will start with a "you are" statement

4. The belief I now have about myself is "I am_____."

    a. The belief will start with an "I am" statement

5. This reminds me of when... (Tell the story of the first time you felt this emotion, thought this meaning, and held this belief about yourself. This will be from your childhood.)

    _____

    _____

    _____

    _____

6. Now connect the dots between the emotion, the meaning, and what you believe about yourself today when this old HURT gets triggered:

    _____

_____

_____

_____

7. Take a moment and forgive yourself for making this up about yourself, and identify the behavior you adopted as a child to deal with HURT of this nature. "I realize that when _____ happens and I feel _____, I believe _____ and then I _____" (what is the behavior you do?).

8. Now reclaim your current age, moving out of the realm of upset child: "I forgot who you really are." Think of the higher Self essence of the person who hurt you. Remember that like you, they too are a spiritual being having a human experience and sometimes get tripped up by the ego. "You are _____."

9. Now reclaim who you are at your core, beyond your ego: "And I forgot who I am." Think of the higher Self essence of you as a spiritual being having a human experience who just had your ego triggered. "I am _____."

10. Reframe your experience to take the learning from it. What shadow aspect of your ego was just mirrored back to you that you can now see thanks to this person who hurt you?

_____

_____

_____

11. How have you hurt others in this same way but with different behaviors?

_____

_____

_____

If people you have hurt are available for a healing conversation, you could take this opportunity to ask for forgiveness. If this is not someone who is safe or someone not available any longer, just ask in proxy. "Will you please forgive me for _____?"

12. Now forgive yourself for taking on this hurt and owning it as yours and for any hurt you have perpetrated on another.

13. Now list what you are grateful for with this experience and how you have grown:

_____

_____

_____

The world is transformed by transformed people. Be willing to self-confront so you can transform the rigidity of mind and body that leads to autoimmune disease into vitality and health that allows you to be the best version of yourself possible.

Next Steps

Whether you have a diagnosed autoimmune illness or are just working on one, my mission is to help you solve your health puzzle. The more people who are healed, the more luminaries we will have to contribute to the world and each other in meaningful ways. The autoimmune puzzle is a complex puzzle; it's not a simple wooden block puzzle that toddlers learn to solve. This is an adult puzzle that requires focused attention and lots of willingness to explore places you might not have ever dreamt you would explore, the labyrinth of your mind and heart.

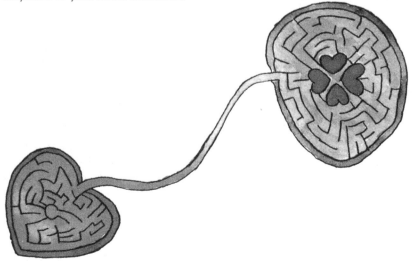

However, you now have a great framework for solving your puzzle. You know the Freedom Framework that builds up the edges; you know the corner pieces that snap in and connect the frame. You know how to alter the picture in the middle by using the 5 R's of healing, and you know the centerpiece that will bring you to your highest Self and closer to your true nature than anything else: forgiveness.

All of this takes practice. You might have found that some of the steps to putting your puzzle together are too difficult for you, that your puzzle is a bit too complex. If that is the case, you can join the other women in the You Un-Broken Program and take it step by step with recorded videos, material, worksheets, guided meditation and interaction with me as part of your community. You might want to start with the Quick Start Program and receive 21 days of emails that provide some tips for getting started on the road to freedom from autoimmunity and then join the WILD Program for some individualized whole life detoxification. If what you have read inspires you to help others heal, then join the other passionate integrative medicine health coaches at the Academy For Integrative Medicine health coach certification program. The world needs more people teaching this work. You can register for the next enrollment in the Resources Section of this book.

You might have gotten all you need in this book and are well on your way to solving your autoimmune puzzle and transforming your autoimmune mindset. Whatever your next step, I am honored to have been on your path with you and wish you infinite blessings and endless joy.

Love and Light,
Dr. Keesha

The End

Resources

The 21 Day Quick Start Program: 21 days of emails that get you started on living a vitality filled life. I will send you my favorite strategies, ideas, products I use myself, recipes, and lots of encouragement. Plus, you will be added to our Woman's Vitality private Facebook community. You can register here: https://drkeesha1.leadpages.co/21-day-quick-start-opt-in-email-series/

The You Un-Broken Online Program and private Facebook community: This incredible program consists of me guiding you through videos, worksheets, and audio recordings through a trauma healing program for emotional freedom. Make sure you know that you might also need a therapist. This program gives you the tools you need to become attuned and aware of your emotional world and will help you stay that way in spite of the inevitable stressful situations in your life. This program is part of the Whole Individualized Life Detox (Wild) Program. When you buy the WILD program, you do not need to purchase the You Un-Broken program.

You can register here: https://drkeesha1.leadpages.co/you-un-broken-online-program/

The Whole Individualized Life Detox (WILD) Online Program and private Facebook community:
The WILD Woman program is the most comprehensive detox program I have ever seen. I have taken all 30 years of my medical training and my certifications and knowledge about the body and how it works into this program. The reason I call it Whole Life is because it works on helping you detox all aspects of your life, not just your liver and your colon. Those are included in this program, but so are the other aspects of your life. It includes the You Un-Broken course because I want to make sure you are well on your way to detoxing your emotional blocks and toxicity.

Then you move into Dr. Keesha's 3 Step Program for Healing Your Hormones, Your Gut and Your Body from the Inside Out.

This program is based on the three-part formula for health:

Your Genetics + Your Exposure to Toxins (physical, emotional, mental, and spiritual) + Your Ability and Willingness to Detox those Toxins = Your Vitality Level

Detoxing is removing what doesn't work so we can replace it with something that does-creating wholeness and vitality.

You will get 5 Modules in 30 Days: You will play with each for 6 days, have a day of rest and integration each week, and then move to the next one. You are in the program for as long as you want to be, and part of the private Facebook community forever. There you will find a rockin' group of WILD Women who support and encourage each other.

This is 30 days to slim, sexy and super-charged!

Register here: https://drkeesha1.leadpages.co/wild-online-program/

The Academy for Integrative Medicine health coach certification program:

Register here: https://www.drkeesha.com/integrative-medicine-health-coach-certification-program/register/

The Academy for Integrative Medicine™ (AIM) Health Coach Certification Program enables you to become a practicing Integrative Medicine health coach, regardless of your educational background and training. If you are a passionate advocate for wellness, let's talk!

This 6-month program will give you all you need to start your own practice. If you're already a provider, it will allow you to integrate integrative medicine health coaching into your practice. This is the only coaching program that will teach you to order and interpret laboratory tests (salivary adrenal and hormone testing, complete stool analysis, and food sensitivity testing) PLUS give you psychology tools to help your clients with their emotional blocks so you can confidently guide your clients to achieve optimal health.

The Integrative Medicine Health Coach Certification Program will:

Teach you in-depth principles of wellness that will allow you to guide others to optimal health, including applied:
- Functional Medicine
- Ayurveda
- Nutrition
- Mind-body medicine
- Positive psychology and Sexology
- Legal and business strategies
- Certify you in Dr. Keesha's scientifically proven protocols and methods for achieving emotional freedom and vibrant health.
- Train you in the art and science of health coaching.
- Instruct you in ordering and interpreting Functional Medicine lab tests.
- Teach you how to create individualized diet, supplementation, exercise, and stress-reducing protocols.
- Provide you with mentorship and a referral network to promote your success.

You will be trained to:
- Identify root causes of illness through appropriate Functional Medicine-based lab testing.
- Implement scientifically proven, drug-free, individually tailored protocols.
- Clearly and confidently communicate healing strategies to your clients. Build a successful and rewarding health coaching business.

Register here: https://www.drkeesha.com/integrative-medicine-health-coach-certification-program/register/

Test Don't Guess:

As I mentioned in the book, testing is a vitally important step for reversing inflammation and autoimmune disease. You can get set up with the right tests by making an appointment with one of my team members or by ordering them directly and then making an appointment with one of my team members for the follow up results and individualized health plan: https://www.drkeesha.com/product-category/consults-lab-tests

Make an appointment with Dr. Keesha or her team:
https://www.drkeesha.com/personal-consultations
or email: info@DrKeesha.com.

Dr. Keesha's Stress Busting Tool Kit:

https://www.drkeesha.com/shop/stress-busting-tool-kit

Find Your Ayurvedic Dosha Type:

https://www.drkeesha.com/dosha-assessment

Functional Nutrients Supplement line:

https://www.drkeesha.com/shop

For more information about the ACEs Study:

https://www.cdc.gov/violenceprevention/acestudy

For Cleaning up Your Environment and Pantry
The Environmental Working Group:

http://www.ewg.org

Find a Trauma Release Therapist
Eye Movement Desensitization Re-Programming (EMDR):

http://www.emdria.org/search/custom.asp?id=2337

Brain Spotting:

http://www.brainspottinginternational.org/find-a-therapist/

Heart Centered Hypnotherapy:

http://providers.wellness-institute.org

Dr. Keesha's Recommended Safe Products
Annmarie organic skin care:

https://www.drkeesha.com/annmarie-skin-care/

Sunlighten Infrared Saunas:

https://www.drkeesha.com/sunlighten-sauna/

Natural bristle bath brush:

https://www.drkeesha.com/recommended-products/

Capomo coffee alternative:

https://www.drkeesha.com/capomo/

Addictive Wellness Raw Chocolate:

https://www.addictivewellness.com/?rfsn=502133.568c8

Himalayan Rock Salt Lamp:
https://www.drkeesha.com/recommended-products/

Going Gluten Free
GlutenFreeSociety.org

Bibliography

Introduction

Germolec, D., Kono, D., Pfau, J., Pollard, K. (2012). Animal models used to examine the role of the environment in the development of autoimmune disease: Findings from an NIEHS Expert Panel Workshop. J Autoimmun; doi:1 0.1016/j.jaut.2012.05.020.

Gilbert, K., Rowley, B., Gomez-Acevedo, H., & Blossom, S. (2011). Co-exposure to mercury increases immunotoxicity of trichloroethylene. Toxicol Sci, 119(2):281-292.

HHS (U.S. Department of Health and Human Services Office on Women's Health) Autoimmune Diseases Fact Sheet. [accessed October 23, 2012].

Jiang, C., Zhao, M., Waters, K., & Diaz, M. (2012). Activation-induced deaminase contributes to the antibody-independent role of B cells in the development of autoimmunity. Autoimmunity 45(6):440-448.

Love, L. (2009). Ultraviolet radiation intensity predicts the relative distribution of dermatomyositis and anti-Mi-2 autoantibodies in women. Arthritis Rheum 60(8):2499-2504.

Marchand, L. et al. (2012). Mesothelial cell and anti-nuclear autoantibodies associated with pleural abnormalities in an asbestos exposed population of Libby MT. Toxicol Lett 208(2):168-173.

Miller, E. & Cohen, J. (2001). An integrative theory of prefrontal cortex function. Annual Review of Neuroscience, 24, 167-202.

Miller, F. et al. (2012). Epidemiology of environmental exposures and human autoimmune diseases: Findings from a National Institute of Environmental Health Sciences Expert Panel Workshop. J. Autoimmun; doi:10.1016/j.jaut.2012.05.002 [Online 25 June 2012].

Nyland, J. et al. (2011). Fetal and maternal immune responses to methylmercury exposure: a cross-sectional study. Environ Res 111(4):584-589.

Parks, C. et al. (2012). Childhood socioeconomic factors and perinatal characteristics influence development of rheumatoid arthritis in adulthood. Ann Rheum Dis; doi:10.1136/annrheumdis-2011-201083.

Satoh, M. et al. (2012). Prevalence and sociodemographic correlates of antinuclear antibodies in the United States. Arthritis Rheum 64(7):2319-2327.

Selmi, C. et al. (2012). Mechanisms of environmental influence on human autoimmunity: A national institute of environmental health sciences expert panel workshop. J Autoimmun; doi:10.1016/j.jaut.2012.05.007.

Chapter 1: My Personal Puzzle

Cooper, G. & Stroehla, B. (2003). The epidemiology of autoimmune diseases. Autoimmun Rev. May;2(3):119-25.

Fairweather, D. & Rose, N. (2004). Women and Autoimmune Diseases. International Conference on Women and Infectious Diseases (ICWID). Volume 10 (11).

Lerner, A., Jeremias, P., & Matthias2, T. (2015). The World Incidence and Prevalence of Autoimmune Diseases is Increasing. International Journal of Celiac Disease, Vol. 3, No. 4, pp 151-155.

Mol, S. et al. (2005). Symptoms of post-traumatic stress disorder after non-traumatic events: Evidence from an open population study. British Journal of Psychiatry, 186, 494-499.

Mora, F. et al. (2011). Stress, neurotransmitters, corticosterone and body-brain integration. J. Brain Research, doi:10.1016/j.brainres.2011.12.049.

Chapter 2: The Big Picture

Burns, V., Drayson, M., Ring, C. & Carroll, D. (2002). Perceived stress and psychological well-being are associated with antibody status after meningitis C conjugate vaccination. Psychosomatic Medicine. 64 (6): 963–970.

Cohen, S.; Doyle, W. & Skoner, D. (1999). Psychological stress, cytokine production, and severity of upper respiratory illness. Psychosomatic Medicine. 61 (2): 175–180.

Cohen, S., Tyrrell, D. & Smith, A. (1993). Negative life events, perceived stress, negative affect, and susceptibility to the common cold. Journal of Personality and Social Psychology. 64 (1): 131–140.

Cohen, S. & Williamson, G. (1988). Perceived stress in a probability sample of the United States. In S. Spacapan & S. Oskamp (Eds.), The social psychology of health: Claremont Symposium on Applied Social Psychology (pp. 3-67). Newbury Park, CA: Sage.

Culhane, J. et al. (2001). Maternal stress is associated with bacterial vaginosis in human pregnancy. Maternal and Child Health Journal. 5 (2): 127–134.

Dyck, D., Short, R. & Vitaliano, P. (1999). Predictors of burden and infectious illness in schizophrenia caregivers. Psychosomatic Medicine. 61 (4): 411–419.

Ebrecht, M. et al. (2004). Perceived stress and cortisol levels predict speed of wound healing in healthy male adults. Psychoneuroendocrinology. 29 (6): 798–809.

Epel, E. et al. (2004). Accelerated telomere shortening in response to life stress. Proceedings of the National Academy of Sciences of the United States of America. 101 (49): 17312–17315.

Freeman, J. (2008). Adult celiac disease followed by onset of systemic lupus erythematosus. Journal of Clinical Gastorenterology, 42(3): 252-55.

Garg, A. et al. (2001). Psychological stress perturbs epidermal permeability barrier homeostasis: implications for the pathogenesis of stress-associated skin disorders. Archives of Dermatology. 137 (1): 53–59.

Glaser, R. et al. (1999). Stress-related changes in proinflammatory cytokine production in wounds. Archives of General Psychiatry. 56 (5): 450–456 Grosse, L. et al. (2016). Cytokine levels in major depression are related to childhood trauma but not to recent stressors. Psychoneuroendocrinology,73:24-31.

Holzel, B. et al. (2010). Stress reduction correlates with structural changes in the amygdala. Social Cognitive & Affective Neuroscience. 5 (1): 11–17.

Kahaly, G. & Schuppan, D. (2015). Celiac disease and endocrine autoimmunity. Digestive Diseases, 33(2): 155-61.

Kramer, J., Ledolter, G., Manon & Bayless, M. (2000). Stress and metabolic control in diabetes mellitus: methodological issues and an illustrative analysis. Annals of Behavioral Medicine. 22 (1): 17–28.

Lane, J., Seskevich, J. & Pieper, C. (2007). Brief meditation training can improve perceived stress and negative mood. Alternative Therapies in Health and Medicine. 13 (1): 38–44.

Maes, M. & Van Bockstaele, D. (1999). The effects of psychological stress on leukocyte subset distribution in humans: evidence of immune activation. Neuropsychobiology. 39 (1): 1–9.

Malarkey, W. et al. (1995). Influence of academic stress and season on 24-hour mean concentrations of ACTH, cortisol, and beta-endorphin. Psychoneuroendocrinology. 20 (5): 499–508.

Marcus, M. et al. (2003). Change in Stress Levels Following Mindfulness-based Stress Reduction in a Therapeutic Community. Addictive Disorders & Their Treatment. 2 (3): 63–68.

Marshall, R. & Garakani, A. (2002). Psychobiology of the acute stress response and its relationship to the psychobiology of post-traumatic stress disorder. Psychiatr. Clin. North Am., 25(2): 385-95.

Morley, S. (1993). Vivid memory for everyday pains. Pain, 55, 55-62.

Murray, J., Ehlers, A. & Mayou, R. A. (2002). Dissociation and post-traumatic stress disorder: two prospective studies of road traffic accident survivors. Br Journal Psych, 180, 363-8.

NIH Progress in Autoimmune Diseases Research. in National Institute of Health Publication No. 05-514 (2005).

Pruessner, J., Hellhammer, D. & Kirschbaum, C. (1999). Burnout, perceived stress, and cortisol responses to awakening. Psychosomatic Medicine. 61 (2): 197–204.

Sapolsky, R. (2004). Why zebras don't get ulcers. New York, NY., Holt Paperbacks.

Schnabel, R. & Kydd, R. (2012). Neuropsychological assessment of distractibility in mild traumatic brain injury and depression. Clin. Neuropsychol., 26(5):769-89.

Schwartz, C. et al., (2003). Differential amygdalar response to novel versus newly familiar neutral faces: a functional MRI probe developed for studying inhibited temperament. Biological Psychiatry, 53(10): 854-862.

Selye, H. (1975). Implications of the stress concept. New York State Journal of Medicine, 75, 2139-2145.

Shewchuk et al. (1999). Trait Influences on Stress Appraisal and Coping: An Evaluation of Alternative Frameworks. Journal of Applied Social Psychology. 29 (4): 685–704.

Stojanovich, L. (2010). Stress and autoimmunity. Autoimmune Rev., 9(5): A271-6.

Stone, A., Mezzacappa, E., Donatone, B. & Gonder, M. (1999). Psychosocial stress and social support are associated with prostate-specific antigen levels in men: results from a community screening program. Health Psychology. 18 (5): 482–486.

Taylor, J. (2015). Psychometric analysis of the Ten-Item Perceived Stress Scale. Psychological Assessment. 27 (1): 90–101.

Wittling, W. (1997). The right hemisphere and the human stress response. Acta. Physiol. Scand., 640, 55-59.

Van Eck, M. & Nicolson, N. (1994). Perceived stress and salivary cortisol in daily life. Annals of Behavioral Medicine. 16 (3): 221–227.

Chapter 3: Sorting the Pieces of the Puzzle

Bland, J. (2017). Defining Function in the Functional Medicine Model. Integr Med (Encinitas). Feb;16(1):22-25.

Flores, M. (2013). P4 medicine: how systems medicine will transform the healthcare sector and society. Per Med. 10(6):565-576.

Gregory, R. (2004). The Blind Leading the Sighted: An Eye-Opening Experience of the Wonders of Perception (PDF). Nature. 430 (7002): 836. doi:10.1038/430836a. PMID 15318199.

Necker, L. (1832). Observations on some remarkable optical phaenomena seen in Switzerland; and on an optical phaenomenon which occurs on viewing a figure of a crystal or geometrical solid. London and Edinburgh Philosophical Magazine and Journal of Science. 1 (5): 329–337.

Panskepp, J. & Biven, L. (2012). The archaeology of Mind: Neuroevolutionary origins of human emotions. New York, NY.: Norton.

Panskepp, J. (1998) Affective neuroscience: The foundations of human and animal emotions. New York, NY.: Oxford University Press.

Pascual-Leone, A., Amedi, A., Fregni, F. & Merabet, L. (2005). The plastic human brain cortex. Annual Review of Neuroscience, 28, 377-401.

Patil, N., Venkatarathnamma, P. & RamchandraRao, S. (2016). Yoga for Lifestyle Diseases. J Ayurveda Integr Med. Oct - Dec;7(4):261-262.

Pearlman, L. A., & Courtois, C. A. (2005). Clinical applications of the attachment framework: Relational treatment of complex trauma. Journal of Traumatic Stress, 18(5), 449-459.

Rifkin, J. (2009). The empathic civilization: The race to global consciousness in a world in crisis. New York, NY.: Tarcher-Penguin Books.

Rilling, F. et al., (2002). A neural basis for social cooperation. Neuron, 35(2): 395-405.

Rusbult, C. & Van Lange, P. (2003). Interdependence, interaction, and relationships. Annual Review of Psychology, 54, 351-375.

Zenner, H. (2017). Individual Biomarkers Using Molecular Personalized Medicine Approaches. ORL J Otorhinolaryngol Relat Spec. Feb 24;79(1-2):7-13. doi: 10.1159/000455811. [Epub ahead of print].

Chapter 4: Trauma

Briere, J., Hodges, M. & Godbout, N. (2010). Traumatic stress, affect dysregulation, and dysfunctional avoidance: A structural equation model. Journal of Traumatic Stress, 23(6):767-774.

Briere, J. & Scott, C. (2007). Assessment of trauma symptoms in eating-disordered populations. Eating Disorders: The Journal of Treatment and Prevention, 15, 1-12.

Briere, J., Scott, C., & Weathers, F.W. (2005). Peritraumatic and persistent dissociation in the presumed etiology of PTSD. American Journal of Psychiatry, 162, 2295-2301.

Briere, J., & Jordan, C.E. (2004). Violence against women: Outcome complexity and implications for treatment. Journal of Interpersonal Violence, 19, 1252-1276.

Briere, J., & Runtz, M.R. (2002). The Inventory of Altered Self-Capacities (IASC): A standardized measure of identity, affect regulation, and relationship disturbance. Assessment, 9, 230-239.

Briere, J., & Rickards, S. (2007). Self-awareness, affect regulation, and relatedness: Differential sequels of childhood versus adult victimization experiences. Journal of Nerv and Mental Disease, 195, 497-503.

Cerqueira, J., Almeida, O. & Sousa, N. (2008). The stressed prefrontal cortex. Left? Right!. Brain, Behavior, and Immunity, 22, 630-638.

Chen Z, Williams KD, Fitness J, Newton NC. (2008). When hurt will not heal: exploring the capacity to relive social and physical pain. Psychol Sci., 19(8), 789-95.

Chu, J.A. & Dill, D.L. (1990). Dissociative symptoms in relation to childhood physical and sexual abuse. Am J Psychiatry, 147(7): 887-892.

Chudakov, B., Cohen, H., Matar, M., & Kaplan, Z. (2008). A naturalistic prospective open study of the effects of adjunctive therapy of sexual dysfunction in chronic PTSD patients. Isr J Psychiatry Relat Sci, 45(1): 26-32.

Ciechanowski, P., Sullivan, M., Jensen, M., Romano, J. & Summers, H. (2003). The relationship of attachment style to depression, catastrophizing and health care utilization in patients with chronic pain. Pain, 104, 627-637.

Clum, G., Calhoun, K., & Kimerling, R. (2000). Associations among symptoms of depression and posttraumatic stress disorder and self-reported health in sexually assaulted women. J Nerv Ment Dis, 188(10):671-8.

Davidson, R. (2013). The emotional life of your brain: How its unique patterns affect the way you think, feel, and live-and how you can change them. New York, NY.: Plume.

Davidson, R. (1998). Anterior electrophysiological asymmetries, emotion, and depression: conceptual and methodological conundrums. Psychophysiology 35, 607-614.

Delahanty, D. L., Raimonde, A. J., Spoonster, E. & Cullado, M. (2003). Injury severity, prior trauma history, urinary cortisol levels, and acute PTSD in motor vehicle accident victims. Journal of Anxiety Disorders, 17, 149-164.

Depue, R. & Morrone-Stupinsky, J. (2005). A neurobehavioral model of affiliative bonding: Implications for conceptualizing a human trait of affiliation. Behavioral and Brain Sciences, 28, 313-350.

Derryberry, D. & Reed, M. (1994). Temperament and attention: Orienting toward and away from positive and negative signals. Journal of Personality and Social Psychology, 66, 1128-1139.

Dube, S. et al. (2009). Cumulative childhood stress and autoimmune diseases in adults. Psychosom Med. 71(2):243-50.

Eccleston, C. & Crombez, G. (1999). Pain demands attention: a cognitive-affective model of the interruptive function of pain. Psychological Bulletin, 125, 356-366.

Eisenberger, N. & Gable, S. (2004). Individual differences in social distress cognitions following conflict. Unpublished data.

Eisenberger, N. & Leiberman, M. (2004). Why rejection hurts: The neurocognitive overlap between physical and social pain. Trends in Cognitive Sciences, 8, 294-300.

Eisenberger, N. et al., (2005). Personality from a controlled processing perspective: An fMRI study of neuroticism, extraversion, and self-consciousness. Cognitive, Affective, & Behavioral Neuroscience, 5(2), 169-181.

Elzinga, B. M. et al. (2003). Higher cortisol levels following exposure to traumatic reminders in abuse-related PTSD. Neuropsychopharmacology, 28, 1656-1665.

Green, B. (2003). Post-traumatic stress disorder: symptom profiles in men and women. Curr med Res Opin., 19(3):200-4.

Green, B., et al. (2001). Psychological outcomes associated with traumatic loss in a sample of young women. American Behavioral Scientist, 44, 817-837.

Grimm, S. et al. (2008). Imbalance between left and right dorsolateral prefrontal cortex in major depression is linked to negative emotional judgment: an fMRI study in severe major depressive disorder. Biological Psychiatry, 63(4):369-376.

Gunthert, K., Cohen, L. & Armeli, S. (1999). The role of neuroticism in daily stress and coping. Journal of Personality and Social Psychology, 77, 1087-1100.

Handwerger-Brohawn, K., Offringa, R., Pfaff, D., Hughes, K., & Shin, L. (2010). The neural correlates of emotional memory in posttraumatic stress disorder. Biological Psychiatry, 68(11):1023-1030.

Hansson, R., Jones, W., & Fletcher, W. (1990). Troubled relationships later in life: implications for support. Journal of Social and Personal Relationships, 7, 451-463.

Howell, A. & Conway, M. (1992). Mood and suppression of positive and negative self-referent thoughts. Cognitive Therapy and Research, 16, 535-555.

Hoyt, W. T., Fincham, F. D., McCullough, M. E., Maio, G., & Davila, J. (2005). Responses to interpersonal transgressions in families: Forgivingness, forgivability, and relationship-specific effects. Journal of Personality and Social Psychology, 89, 375-394.

Javidi, H. & Yadollahie, M. (2012). Post-traumatic stress disorder. Int J Occup Environ Med., 3(1):2-9.

Johnstone, T., van Reekum, C., Urry, H., Kalin, N. & Davidson, R. (2007). Failure to regulate: counterproductive recruitment of top-down prefrontal-subcortical circuitry in major depression. J. Neurosci., 27, 8877-84.

Jung, C. G. (1969). On the nature of the psyche. Princeton, N.J.: Princeton University Press.

Kagan, J., Reznick, J. & Gibbons, J. (1989). Inhibited and uninhibited types of children. Child Development, 60, 838-45.

Kagan, J., Schwartz, C., Wright, C., Shin, J. and Rauch, S. (2003). Inhibited and uninhibited infants grown up: Adult amygdalar response to novelty. Science, 300, 1952-53.

Lukaschek, K. et al. (2012). Lifetime traumatic experiences and their impact on PTSD: a general population study. Soc. Psychiatry Psychiatr Epidemiol., doi: 10.1007/s00127-012-0585-7.

Mendola, R., Tennen, H., Affleck, G., McCann, L., and Fitzgerald, T. (1990). Appraisal and adaptation among women with impaired fertility. Cognitive Therapy and Research, 14, 79-93.

Mickley-Steinmetz, K., Scott, L., Smith, D. & Kensinger, E. (2012). The effects of trauma exposure and posttraumatic stress disorder (PTSD) on the emotion-induced memory trade-off. Front Integr Neurosci., 6: 34.

Mickley-Steinmetz, K. & Kensinger, E. (2012). The emotion-induced memory trade-off: more than an effect of overt attention? doi:10.3758/s13421-012-0247-8.

Levine, P. (2010). In an Unspoken Voice: How the Body Releases Trauma and Restores Goodness. Berkley, CA.: North Atlantic.

Panasetis, P. & Bryant, R. (2003). Peritraumatic versus persistent dissociation in acute stress disorder. Journal of Traumatic Stress, 16(6):563-66.

Rothschild, B. (2000). The body remembers: The psychophysiology of trauma and trauma treatment. New York, NY.: Norton.

Shapiro, F. (2012). Getting Past Your Past: Take Control of Your Life with Self-Help Techniques from EMDR Therapy. New York, NY.: Rodale.

Van der Kolk, B. (2014). The Body Keeps the Score: Brain, Mind, and Body in the Healing of Trauma. New York, NY.: Penguin.

Van der Kolk, M. et al. (1996). Dissociation, Affect Dysregulation & Somatization: the complex nature of adaptation to trauma. American Journal of Psychiatry, 153(7):183-93.

Vaughn, G. S. & Dowdy, S.W. (2005) Development and validation of the emotional intimacy scale. Journal of Nursing Measurement, 13(3), 193-206.

Waring, J.D. & Kensinger, E. (2011). How emotion leads to selective memory: neuroimaging evidence. Neuropsychologia, 49(7):1831-42.

Watson, D. & Pennebaker, J. (1989). Health complaints, stress, and distress: exploring the central role of negative affectivity. Psychological Review, 96, 234-254.

Chapter 5: Leaky Gut

Akbari, P. et al. (2016). The intestinal barrier as an emerging target in the toxicological assessment of mycotoxins. Arch Toxicol.

Arrieta, M. et al. (2006). Alterations in intestinal permeability. Gut. 55(10):1512-20.

Bischoff, S. et al. (2014). Intestinal permeability--a new target for disease prevention and therapy. BMC Gastroenterol (Review). 14: 189. doi:10.1186/s12876-014-0189-7.

Csaki, K. (2011). Synthetic surfactant food additives can cause intestinal barrier dysfunction. Medical Hypotheses, 76(5): 676-81.

Daulatzai, M. (2015). Non-celiac gluten sensitivity triggers gut dysbiosis, neuroinflammation, gut-brain axis dysfunction, and vulnerability for dementia. CNS and Neurological Disorders: Drug Targets, 14(1): 110-31.

DePunder, K. & Pruimboom, L. (2013). The dietary intake of wheat and other cereal grains and their role in inflammation. Nutrients, 5(3): 771-87.

Drago, S. et al. (2006). Gliadin, zonulin and gut permeability: Effects on celiac and non-celiac intestinal mucosa and intestinal cell lines. Scand J Gastroenterol. 41(4):408-19.

Fasano, A. (2012) Leaky gut and autoimmune diseases. Clin Rev Allergy Immunol. Feb;42(1):71-8.

Fasano, A. et al. (2015). Non-celiac gluten sensitivity. Gastroenterology. 148(6): 1195-204.

Fasano, A. (2011). Zonulin and its regulation of intestinal barrier function: the biological door to inflammation, autoimmunity, and cancer. Physiol Rev. 91(1):151-75.

Gecse, K. et al. (2012). Leaky gut in patients with diarrhea-predominant irritable bowel syndrome and inactive ulcerative colitis. Digestion. 85(1):40-6.

Gershon, M. (1998). The Second Brain: A Groundbreaking New Understanding of the Nervous Disorders of the Stomach and Intestine. New York: Harper Collins.

Hartwell, K. et al. (2013); Association of elevated cytokines with childhood adversity in a sample of healthy adults. J. Psychiatric Res., 47(5):604-10.

Hollander, D. (1999). Intestinal permeability, leaky gut, and intestinal disorders. Curr Gastroenterol Rep. 1(5):410-6.

Humbert, P. et al. (1991). Intestinal permeability in patients with psoriasis. Journal of dermatological science 2 (4): 324–326.

Khalif, I., et al. (2005). Alterations in the colonic flora and intestinal permeability and evidence of immune activation in chronic constipation. Dig Liver Dis. 7:838–49.

Kiefer, D., Ali-Akbarian L (2004). A brief evidence-based review of two gastrointestinal illnesses: irritable bowel and leaky gut syndromes. Alternative Therapy Health Medicine 10 (3): 22–30.

Klingensmith, N. & Coopersmith, C. (2016). The Gut as the Motor of Multiple Organ Dysfunction in Critical Illness. Crit Care Clin (Review). 32 (2): 203–12.

Liu, Z. et al. (2005). Tight junctions, leaky intestines, and pediatric diseases. Acta Paediatr. 94(4):386-93.

NHS Choices (2015). Leaky gut syndrome. Retrieved 15 August 2016.

Lee, S. (2015). Intestinal permeability regulation by tight junction: Implication on inflammatory bowel diseases. Intestinal Research, 13(1): 11-18.

Lerner, A. & Matthias, T. (2015). Changes in intestinal tight junction permeability associated with industrial food additives explain the rising incidence of autoimmune disease. Autoimmunity Reviews, 14(6): 479-89.

Liu, Z., Li, N., Neu, J. (2005). Tight junctions, leaky intestines, and pediatric diseases, Acta Paediatrica , 94(4), pp. 386-393.

Maes, M., Leunis, J. (2008). Normalization of leaky gut in chronic fatigue syndrome (CFS) is accompanied by a clinical improvement: effects of age, duration of illness and the translocation of LPS from gram-negative bacteria, Journal of Neuro Endocrinology, 29(6), pp. 902-10.

Maes, M. et al. (2008). The gut-brain barrier in major depression: intestinal mucosal dysfunction with an increased translocation of LPS from gram negative enterobacteria (leaky gut) plays a role in the inflammatory pathophysiology of depression. Neuro Endocrinol Lett. 29(1):117-24.

Mezzelani, A. et al. (2014). Environment, dysbiosis, immunity and sex-specific susceptibility: A translational hypothesis for regressive autism pathogenesis. Nutr Neurosci. [Epub ahead of print]

Mitchell, N. (2011). Randomized controlled trial of food elimination diet based on IgG antibodies for the prevention of migraine like headaches. Nutritional Journal, 10(8).

Odenwald, M. & Turner, J. (2013). Intestinal Permeability Defects: Is It Time to Treat? Clinical Gastroenterology and Hepatology. 11 (9): 1075–83.

Pike, M. et al. (1986). Increased Intestinal Permeability in Atopic Eczema. Journal of Investigative Dermatology 86 (2): 101–104.

Powley, T. and Phillips, R. (2002). Morphology and topography of vagal afferents innervating the GI tract. American Journal of Physiology: Gastrointestinal and Liver Physiology. 283(6); G1217-25.

Rao, M. & Gershon, M. (2016). The bowel and beyond: the enteric nervous system in neurological disorders. Nat Rev Gastroenterol Hepatol (Review). 13 (9): 517–28.

Sanz, Y. (2010). Effects of gluten free diet on gut microbiota and immune function in healthy adult humans. Gut Microbes, 1(3): 135-37.

Takeuchi, K. & Satoh, H. (2015). NSAID-induced small intestinal damage-roles of various pathogenic factors. Digestion, 91(3): 218-32.

Troncone, R. & Discepolio, V. (2014). Celiac disease and autoimmunity. Journal of Pediatric Gastroenterology and Nutrition. 59(1): S9-S11.

Vaarala, O., Atkinson, M., Neu, J. (2008). The "Perfect Storm" for Type 1 Diabetes The Complex Interplay Between Intestinal Microbiota, Gut Permeability, and Mucosal Immunity', Diabetes Journal, (57)10(2555-2562).

Visser, J. (2010). Tight Junctions, Intestinal Permiability and Autoimmunity Celiac Disease and Type 1 Diabetes Paradigms. PubMed.

Weinstock, L. & Walters, A. (2011). Restless legs syndrome is associated with irritable bowel syndrome and small intestinal bacterial overgrowth. Sleep Medicine. 12(6): 610-613.

Yarandi, S. et al. (2016). Modulatory Effects of Gut Microbiota on the Central Nervous System: How Gut Could Play a Role in Neuropsychiatric Health and Diseases. J Neurogastroenterol Motil (Review). 22 (2): 201–12.

Chapter 6: Environmental Toxicity

Breeding, P., Russell, N. & Nicolson, G. (2012). An integrative model of chronically activated immune-hormonal pathways important in the generation of fibromyalgia. British Journal of Medical Practitioners, 5(3): a524-a534.

Calafat, A.,Ye, X., Wong, L., Bishop, A. & Needham, L. (2010). Urinary concentrations of four parabens in the U.S. population: NHANES 2005-2006. Environ Health Perspect. 118(5):679-85.

http://www.cas.org/content/chemical-substances

https://www.cdc.gov/epstein-barr/about-ebv.html

https://www.drugabuse.gov/publications/drusgfacts/drug-related-hospital-emergency-room-visits

EFSA. (2004). Opinion of the Scientific Panel on food additives, flavourings, processing aids and materials in contact with food (AFC) related to para hydroxybenzoates (E 214-219). EFSA Journal. 83, 1-26.

https://www.endocrinescience.org/principles-for-identifying-endocrine-active-and-endocrine-disrupting-chemicals/?gclid=CM6hkoOh-dECFYdbfgodsYsJBA

http://www.ewg.org/guides/cleaners

http://www.ewg.org/skindeep/

http://www.fda.gov/Drugs/DevelopmentApprovalProcess/DevelopmentResources/DrugInteractionsLabeling/ucm110632.htm

Jacubeit, T., Drisch, D., & Weber, E. (1990). Risk factors as reflected by an intensive drug monitoring system. Agents Actions, 29:117–125.

Junker, Y. et al. (2012). Wheat amylase trypsin inhibitors drive intestinal inflammation via activation of toll-like receptor 4. Journal of Experimental Medicine, 209(13): 2395-408.

Mehrpour, O. et al. (2014). Occupational exposure to pesticides and consequences on male semen and fertility: a review. Toxicology Letters. 230(2): 146-56.

Molina, V. & Shoenfeld, Y. (2005) Infection, vaccines and other environmental triggers of autoimmunity. Autoimmunity, 38(3):235-45.

Nicolson, G. & Haier, J. (2009). Role of Chronic Bacterial and Viral Infections in Neurodegenerative, Neurobehavioral, Psychiatric, Autoimmune and Fatiguing Illnesses: Part 1, British Journal of Medical Practitioners; 2(4): 20-28.

Nicolson, G. & Haier, J. (2010). Role of Chronic Bacterial and Viral Infections in Neurodegenerative, Neurobehavioral, Psychiatric, Autoimmune and Fatiguing Illnesses: Part 2, British Journal of Medical Practitioners; 3(1): 301-311.

Nicolson, G. (2008). Chronic Bacterial and Viral Infections in Neurodegenerative and Neurobehavioral Diseases. Laboratory Medicine, 39(5): 291-299.

https://www.nrdc.org/stories/9-ways-avoid-hormone-disrupting-chemicals?gclid=CPSdls-Wh-dECFQ-dfgodYa0Dfg.

Oishi, S. (2002). Effects of propyl paraben on the male reproductive system. Food Chem Toxicol. Dec; 40(12):1807-13.

Routledge, E. et al. (1998). Some alkyl hydroxy benzoate preservatives (parabens) are estrogenic. Toxicol Appl Pharmacol. 153(1):12-9.

Roy, D. et al. (1997). Biochemical and molecular changes at the cellular level in response to exposure to environmental estrogen-like chemicals. Journal of Toxicology and Environmental Health, 50(1): 1-29.

Schuppan, D. & Zevallos, V. (2015). Wheat amylase trypsin inhibitors as nutritional activators of innate immunity. Digestive Diseases, 33(2): 260-63.

Smith, K. (2013). Urinary paraben concentrations and ovarian aging among women from a fertility center. Environ Health Perspect. 121(11-12):1299-305.

Teixeira, D. et al. (2015). Inflammatory and cardiometabolic risk on obesity: role of environmental xenoestrogens. Journal of Clinical Endocrinology & Metabolism, 100(5): 1792-801.

Terasaka, S., Inoue, A., Tanji, M., & Kiyama, R. (2006). Expression profiling of estrogen-responsive genes in breast cancer cells treated with alkylphenols, chlorinated phenols, parabens, or bis- and benzoylphenols for evaluation of estrogenic activity. Toxicol Lett. 163(2):130-41. Epub 2005 Nov 8.

Triggs, C. et al. (2010). Dietary factors in chronic inflammation: food tolerances and intolerances of a New Zealand Caucasian Crohn's disease population. Mutation Research/Fundamental and Molecular Mechanisms of Mutagenesis. 690(1): 123-38.

Vo, T. et al. (2011). Estrogen receptor α is involved in the induction of Calbindin-D(9k) and progesterone receptor by parabens in GH3 cells: a biomarker gene for screening xenoestrogens. Steroids. 76(7):675-81.

Vojdani, A. et al. (2014). Environmental triggers and autoimmunity. Autoimmune disease.

Watson, C. et al. (2014). Rapid actions of xenoestrogens disrupt normal estrogenic signaling. Steroids, 81: 36-42.

Wróbel, A. & Gregoraszczuk, E. (2014). Actions of methyl-, propyl- and butylparaben on estrogen receptor-α and -β and the progesterone receptor in MCF-7 cancer cells and non-cancerous MCF-10A cells. Toxicol Lett. 230(3):375-381

Chapter 7: Genetics

Arbuckle, M. et al. (2003). Development of autoantibodies before the clinical onset of systemic lupus erythematosus. N Engl J Med. 349:1526-1533.

Aune, T. (2004). Gene expression profiles in human autoimmune disease. Program and abstracts of the 54th Annual Meeting of the American Society of Human Genetics; October 26-30, 2004; Toronto, Ontario, Canada.

Aune, T., Maas, K., Moore, J., & Olsen, N. (2003). Gene expression profiles in human autoimmune disease. Curr Pharm Des. 9:1905-1917.

Aune, T. et al. (2004). Co-localization of differentially expressed genes and shared susceptibility loci in human autoimmunity. Genet Epidemiol. 27:162-172.

Auxemery, Y. (2012). Post-traumatic stress disorder as a consequence of the interaction between an individual genetic susceptibility, a traumatogenic event and a social context. Encephale, 38(5):373-80.

Baechler, E. et al. (2004). Expression levels for many genes in human peripheral blood cells are highly sensitive to ex vivo incubation. Genes Immun. 5:347-353.

Barreiro, L. (2008). Natural selection has driven population differentiation in modern humans. Nat. Genet. 40, 340–345.

Barreiro, L. & Quintana-Murci, L. (2010). From evolutionary genetics to human immunology: how selection shapes host defense genes. Nat. Rev. Genet. 11, 17–30.

Bottini, N. et al. (2004). A functional variant of lymphoid tyrosine phosphatase is associated with type I diabetes. Nat Genet. 36:337-338.

Cantor, R. et al. (2004). Systemic lupus erythematosus genome scan: Support for linkage at 1q23, 2q33, 16q12-13, and 17q21-23 and novel evidence at 3p24, 10q23-24, 13q32, and 18q22-23. Arthritis Rheum. 50:3203-3210.

Carvalheiras, G., Faria, R., Braga, J. & Vasconcelos, C. (2013). Fetal outcome in autoimmune diseases. Autoimmun. Rev. 11, A520–A530.

Ceccarelli, F., Agmon-Levin, N. & Perricone, C. (2016). Genetic Factors of Autoimmune Diseases. Journal of Immunology Research. http://dx.doi.org/10.1155/2016/3476023.

Choudhury, A. et al. (2014). Population-specific common SNPs reflect demographic histories and highlight regions of genomic plasticity with functional relevance. BMC Genomics 15, 437.

Clowse, M. et al. (2012). Effects of infertility, pregnancy loss, and patient concerns on family size of women with rheumatoid arthritis and systemic lupus erythematosus. Arthritis Care Res. 64, 668–674.

Cooper, G., Bynum, M. & Somers, E. (2009). Recent insights in the epidemiology of autoimmune diseases: improved prevalence estimates and understanding of clustering of diseases. J. Autoimmun. 33, 197–207.

Costenbader, K., Gay, S., Alarcón-Riquelme, M., Iaccarino, L. and Doria, A. (2012). Genes, epigenetic regulation and environmental factors: which is the most relevant in developing autoimmune diseases? Autoimmunity Reviews, 11(8): 604–609, 2012.

Ferguson, L. et al. (2007). Nutrigenomics and gut health. Nutrigenomics, 622(1-2).

Fumagalli, M. et al. (2011). Signatures of environmental genetic adaptation pinpoint pathogens as the main selective pressure through human evolution. PLoS Genet. 7, e1002355.

Gregersen, P. (2004). Susceptibility genes in rheumatoid arthritis. Program and abstracts of the 54th Annual Meeting of the American Society of Human Genetics; October 26-30, 2004; Toronto, Ontario, Canada.

Gregersen, P. (2003). Teasing apart the complex genetics of human autoimmunity: lessons from rheumatoid arthritis. Clin Immunol. 107:1-9.

Gregersen, K. & Brehrens, T. (2003). Fine mapping the phenotype in autoimmune disease: the promise and pitfalls of DNA microarray technologies. Genes Immun. 4:175-176.

Haines, J. (2004). Susceptibility loci for multiple sclerosis. Program and abstracts of the 54th Annual Meeting of the American Society of Human Genetics; October 26-30, Toronto, Ontario, Canada.

Jawaheer, D. et al. (2004). Clustering of disease features within 512 multicase rheumatoid arthritis families. Arthritis Rheum. 50:736-741.

Jostins, L. et al. (2012). Host-microbe interactions have shaped the genetic architecture of inflammatory bowel disease. Nature 491, 119–124.

Kenealy, S., Pericak-Vance, M., & Haines, J. The genetic epidemiology of multiple sclerosis. J Neuroimmunol. 143:7-12.

Kyogoku, C. et al. (2004). A missense single-nucleotide polymorphism in a gene encoding a protein tyrosine phosphatase (PTPN22) is associated with rheumatoid arthritis. Am J Hum Genet. 75:330-337.

Kyogoku, C. (2004). Genetic association of the R620W polymorphism of protein tyrosine phosphatase PTPN22 with human SLE. Am J Hum Genet. 75:504-507.

LeDoux, J. (2002). Synaptic self: How our brains become who we are. New York, NY.: Penguin.

Liu, Z., Maas, K., & Aune, T. (2004). Comparison of differentially expressed genes in T lymphocytes between human autoimmune disease and murine models of autoimmune disease. Clin Immunol. 112:225-230.

Maas, K., et al. (2002). Cutting edge: molecular portrait of human autoimmune disease. J. Immunol., 169:5-9.

Mariani, S. (2004). Genes and Autoimmune Diseases -- A Complex Inheritance. Highlights of the 54th Annual Meeting of the American Society of Human Genetics; October 26-30, Toronto, Ontario, Canada. MedGenMed, 6(4): 18.

McGrogan, A., Snowball, J. & de Vries, C. (2014). Pregnancy losses in women with type 1 or type 2 diabetes in the UK: an investigation using primary care records. Diabet. Med. 31, 357–365.

Moore, J., Parker, J., Olsen, N., & Aune, T. (2002). Symbolic discriminant analysis of microarray data in autoimmune disease. Genet Epidemiol. 23:57-69.

Nagy, G., et al. (2015). Selected aspects in the pathogenesis of autoimmune diseases. Mediators of Inflammation.

Neel, J. (2015). Diabetes Mellitus: A thrifty genotype rendered detrimental by progress. Department of Human Genetics, University of Michigan Medical School, Ann Arbor, Michigan.

Okin, D. & Medzhitov, R. (2012). Evolution of inflammatory diseases. Curr. Biol. 22, R733–R740.

Olshansky, S. et al. (2005). A potential decline in life expectancy in the United States in the 21st century. New England Journal of Medicine, 352(11): 1138-45.

Ostensen, M. et al. (2015). State of the art: reproduction and pregnancy in rheumatic diseases. Autoimmun. Rev. 14, 376–386.

Parkes, M., Cortes, A., van Heel, D. A. & Brown, M. A. (2013). Genetic insights into common pathways and complex relationships among immune-mediated diseases. Nat. Rev. Genet. 14, 661–673.

Paula, S. et al. (2015). Genetics of autoimmune diseases: insights from population genetics. Journal of Human Genetics, 60, 657–664.

Perricone, C., Ceccarelli, F., and Valesini, G. (2011). An overview on the genetic of rheumatoid arthritis: a never-ending story. Autoimmunity Reviews, 10(10):599–608.

Quintana-Murci, L. & Clark, A. (2013). Population genetic tools for dissecting innate immunity in humans. Nat. Rev. Immunol. 13, 280–293.

Raj, T. et al. (2013). Common risk alleles for inflammatory diseases are targets of recent positive selection. Am. J. Hum. Genet. 92, 517–529.

Ramos, P. et al. (2011). A comprehensive analysis of shared loci between systemic lupus erythematosus (SLE) and sixteen autoimmune diseases reveals limited genetic overlap. PLoS Genet. 7.

Ramos, P. S., Shaftman, S. R., Ward, R. C. & Langefeld, C. D. (2014). Genes associated with SLE are targets of recent positive selection. Autoimmune Dis.

Ravussin, E. et al. (1994). Effects of a traditional lifestyle on obesity in Pima Indians. Diabetes Care, 17(9): 1067-74.

Roden, D. (2017). Phenome-wide association studies: A new method for functional genomics in humans. J Physiol. Feb 23. doi: 10.1113/JP273122. [Epub ahead of print]

Sawcer, S. et al. (2004). Enhancing linkage analysis of complex disorders: an evaluation of high-density genotyping. Hum Mol Genet. 13:1943-1949.

Selmi, C., Lu, Q. & Humble, M. C. (2012). Heritability versus the role of the environment in autoimmunity. J. Autoimmun. 39, 249–252.

Shen, N. & Tsao, B. (2004). Current advances in the human lupus genetics. Curr Rheumatol Rep. 6:391-398.

Simopoulos, A. (2006). Evolutionary aspects of diet, the omega 6/omega 3 ratio and genetic variation: nutritional implications for chronic diseases. Biomedicine & Pharmacotherapy, 60(9): 502-7.

Strachan, D. (1989). Hay fever, hygiene, and household size. B.M.J. 299, 1259–1260.

Sultan, C. et al. (2001). Environmental xenoestrogens, antiandrogens and disorders of male sexual differentiation. Molecular and Cellular Endocrinology, 178(1-2): 99-105.

Torkamani, A. et al. (2012). Clinical implications of human population differences in genome-wide rates of functional genotypes. Front Genet. 3, 211.

Tsao, B. (2004). The genetics of human systemic lupus erythematosus. Program and abstracts of the 54th Annual Meeting of the American Society of Human Genetics; October 26-30, Toronto, Ontario, Canada.

Tsao, B. (2004). Update on human systemic lupus erythematosus genetics. Curr Opin Rheumatol. 16:513-521.

Van Heemst, J.et al. (2015). Protective effect of HLA-DRB1⬜13 alleles during specific phases in the development of ACPA-positive RA. Annals of the Rheumatic Diseases.

Yurist-Doutsch, S. et al. (2014). Gastrointestinal microbiota-mediated control of enteric pathogens. Annual Review of Genetics, 48: 361-82.

Zhernakova, A. et al. (2010). Evolutionary and functional analysis of celiac risk loci reveals SH2B3 as a protective factor against bacterial infection. Am. J. Hum. Genet.86, 970–977.

Chapter 8: Listening to the Feedback of Your Body

Alter, J. (2004). Yoga in modern India: the body between science and philosophy. Princeton, N.J.: Princeton University Press.

Arikha, N. (2007). Passions and tempers: a history of the humours. New York, NY: Ecco

Atreya (2001). Perfect balance: ayurvedic nutrition for mind, body, and soul. New York: Avery.

Das, R. (2003). The origin of the life of a human being: conception and the female according to ancient Indian medical and sexological literature. Delhi: Motilal Banarsidass Publishers.

Frawley, D. (1997). Ayurveda and the mind: the healing of consciousness. Twin Lakes, Wis.: Lotus Press.

Frawley, D. and Sandra S.K. (2001). Yoga for your type: an Ayurvedic approach to your Asana practice. Twin Lakes, WI: Lotus.

Kacera, W. (2006). Ayurvedic tongue diagnosis. Twin Lakes, Wis.: Lotus Press.

Khalsa, K. P. S. & Tierra, M. (2008). The way of ayurvedic herbs: the most complete guide to natural healing and health with traditional ayurvedic herbalism. Twin Lakes, Wis.: Lotus.

Lad, V. (1984). Ayurveda: the science of self-healing: a practical guide. Santa Fe, N.M.: Lotus Press.

Lad, V. & Frawley, D. (1986). The yoga of herbs: an Ayurvedic guide to herbal medicine. Santa Fe, N.M.: Lotus Press.

Lad, V. (1998). The complete book of Ayurvedic home remedies. New York: Harmony Books.

Lad, V. (2012). Textbook of Ayurveda. Albuquerque, N.M.: Ayurvedic Press.

Lad, V. & Crowther, G. (2005). Ayurvedic perspectives on selected pathologies: an anthology of essential reading from ayurveda today. Albuquerque, NM: Ayurvedic Press.

Morningstar, A. & Desai, U. (1990). The Ayurvedic cookbook: a personalized guide to good nutrition and health. Santa Fe, NM: Lotus Press.

Pole, S. (2013). Ayurvedic medicine: the principles of traditional practice. London: Singing Dragon.

Ranade, S. & Frawley, D. (1999). Natural healing through Ayurveda. Delhi: Motilal Banarsidass Publishers Private Limited.

Ranade, S. & Ranade, S. (2003). Concept of Ayurvedic physiology: (sharira kriya). Pune: R.D. Nandurkar.

Sharma, P. (1981). Caraka-saṃhitā: Agniveśa's treatise refined and annotated by Caraka and redacted by Dṛḍhabala: text with Engl. transl. Varanasi: Chaukhambha Orientalia.

Stiles, M. (2007). Ayurvedic yoga therapy. Twin Lakes, Wis.: Lotus.

Svoboda, R. (1988). Prakriti: your Ayurvedic constitution. Albuquerque, N.M.: GEOCO.

Tiwari, M. (1995). Ayurveda secrets of healing: the complete Ayurvedic guide to healing through Pancha Karma seasonal therapies, diet, herbal remedies, and memory. Twin Lakes, Wis.: Lotus Press.

Wujastyk, D. (2003). The Roots of Ayurveda: selections from Sankskrit medical writings. Rev. ed. London: Penguin Books.

Chapter 9: No One Size Fits All

Brestoff, J. & Artis, D. (2013). Commensal bacteria at the interface of host metabolism and the immune system. Nature Immunology, 14: 676-84.

Caruso, R. et al. (2013). Appropriate nutrient supplementation in celiac disease. Annals of Medicine, 45(8): 522-31.

De Sousa Moraes, L. et al. (2014). Intestinal microbiota and probiotics in celiac disease. Clinical Microbiology Reviews, 27(3): 482-89.

Lamprecht, M. & Frauwallner, A. (2012). Exercise, intestinal barrier dysfunction and probiotic supplementation. Medicine and Sport Science: Acute Topics in Sport Nutrition, 59: 47-56.

Ley, R. et al. (2006). Microbial ecology: human gut microbes associated with obesity. Nature, 444(7122): 1022-23.

Olivares, M. et al. (2014). Double blind randomized, placebo controlled intervention trial to evaluate the effects of bifidobacterium longum CECT 7347 in children with newly diagnosed celiac disease. British Journal of Nutrition, 112(1): 30-40.

Pickett-Blakely, O. (2014). Obesity and irritable bowel syndrome: a comprehensive review. Gastroenterology and Hepatology, 10(7): 411-16.

Sanz, Y. (2011). Unraveling the ties between celiac disease and intestinal microbiota. International Reviews of Immunology, 30(4): 207-18.

Song, S. et al. (2015). Metabolic syndrome risk factors are associated with white rice intake in Korean adolescent girls and boys. British Journal of Nutrition, 113(3): 479-87.

Vazquez-Roque, M. et al. (2013). A controlled trial of gluten free diet in patients with irritable bowel syndrome diarrhea: effects on bowel frequency and intestinal function. Gastroenterology, 144(5): 903-11.

Zuhl, M. (2014). Effects of oral glutamine supplementation on exercise-induced gastrointestinal permeability and tight junction protein expression. Journal of Applied Physiology, 116(2): 183-91.

Zuniga, Y. et al. (2014). Rice and noodle consumption is associated with insulin resistance and hyperglycemia in an Asian population. British Journal of Nutrition, 111(6): 1118-28.

Chapter 10: Finding Your HURT

Aardal-Eriksson, E., Eriksson, T. E. & Thorell, L. H. (2001). Salivary cortisol, posstraumatic stress symptoms, and general health in the acute phase and during 9-month follow-up. Biological Psychiatry, 15, 986-993.

Becker, J., Skinner, L., Abel, G., & Cichon, J. (1986). Level of post-assault sexual functioning in rape and incest victims. Arch. Sex. Behav., 15:37-49.

Bell, D. & Esses, V. (1997). Ambivalence and response amplification toward negative peoples. Journal of Applied Social Psychology, 27, 1063-1084.

Bolger, N., DeLongis, A., Kessler, R. & Schilling, E. (1989). Effects of daily stress on negative mood. J. Pers. Soc. Psychol., 57(5):808-18.

Damasio, A. (1994). Descartes' Error, Emotion, Reason, and the Human Brain. New York, NY.: Avon Books.

Ford, J. (1999). Disorders of extreme stress following warzone military trauma: associated features of post-traumatic stress disorder (PTSD) or comorbid but distinct syndromes? Journal of Consulting and Clinical Psychology, 67(1), 3-12.

Fox, C. & Halbrook, B. (1994). Terminating relationships at mid-life: A qualitative investigation of low-income women's experiences. Journal of Mental Health Counseling, 16, 143-154.

Franklin, K., Janoff-Bulman, R., and Roberts, J. (1990). Long-term impact of parental divorce on optimism and trust: Changes in general assumptions or narrow beliefs?, Journal of Personality and Social Psychology, 59, 743-755.

Friedman, M., Keane, T. & Resick, P. (eds.) (2007). Handbook of PTSD: science and practice. New York, NY: Guilford Press

Kachadourian, L.K., Fincham, F. & Davila, J. (2005). Attitudinal ambivalence, rumination, and forgiveness of partner transgressions in marriage. Pers Soc Psychol Bull., 31(3), 334-42.

Karney, B., Bradbury, T., Fincham, F., and Sullivan, K. (1994). The role of negative affectivity in the association between attributions and marital satisfaction. Journal of Personality and Social Psychology, 66, 413-424.

Katz, I. & Hass, R. (1988). Racial ambivalence and American value conflict: correlational and priming studies of dual cognitive structures. Journal of Personality and Social Psychology, 55, 893-905.

Keen, S. (1986). Faces of the enemy: Reflections of the hostile imagination. San Francisco, CA.: Harper and Row.

Kiecolt-Glazer, J. et al. (1993). Negative behavior during marital conflict is associated with immunological down-regulation. Psychosomatic Medicine, 55, 395-409.

McCormick, R., Dowd, E., Quirk, S. & Zegatta, J. (1998). The relationship of NEO-PI performance to coping styles, patterns of use, and triggers for use among substance abusers. Addictive Behaviors, 23, 497-507.

McCullough, M. E., Emmons, R. A., Kilpatrick, S. D., & Mooney, C. N. (2003). Narcissists as "victims": The role of narcissism in the perception of transgressions. Personality and Social Psychology Bulletin, 29, 885-893.

Porter, S. & Peace, K. (2007). The scars of memory: a prospective, longitudinal investigation of the consistency of traumatic and positive emotional memories in adulthood. Psychological Science, 18, 435-441.

Santa Maria, A., Reichert, F. & Hummel, S. (2012). Effects of rumination on intrusive memories: does processing mode matter? Journal of Behavior Therapy and Experimental Psychiatry, 43(3): 901-909.

Suarez, E.C., Harlan, E., Peoples, M.C. & Williams, R.B. Jr. (1993). Cardiovascular and emotional responses in women: the role of hostility and harassment. Health Psychol., 12(6), 459-68.

Sullivan, M. & Conway, M. (1991). Dysphoria and valence of attributions for other's behavior. Cognitive Therapy and Research, 15, 273-282.

Tabak, B. A., & McCullough, M. E. (2011). Perceived transgressor agreeableness decreases cortisol response and increases forgiveness following recent interpersonal transgressions. Biological Psychology (in press).

Tabak, B. A., McCullough, M. E., Szeto, A., Mendez, A. J., McCabe, P. M. (2011). Oxytocin indexes relational distress following interpersonal harms in women. Psychoneuroendocrinology, 36, 115-122.

Taylor, D.J. et al. (2010). Which depressive symptoms remain after response to cognitive therapy of depression and predict relapse and recurrence? J Affect Disord.,123(1-3),181-7.

Chapters 11-15: Healing the HURT

Bono, G. & McCullough M. E. (2006). Positive responses to benefit and harm: Bringing forgiveness and gratitude into cognitive psychotherapy. Journal of Cognitive Psychotherapy, 20, 147-158.

Boszormenyi-Nagy, I. (1986). Contextual therapy and the unity of therapies (pp. 65-72). In J.C. Hansen (ed.), The interface of individual and family therapy. Rockville, MD: Aspen Publications.

Boszormenyi-Nagy, I., Grunebaum, J. & Ulrich, D., (1991). Contextual therapy (pp. 200-238). In A.S. Gurman & D. P. Kniskern (eds.). Handbook of family therapy (Vol. II). New York, NY: Brunner/Mazel.

Bowlby, J. (1969). Attachment & Loss, Vol. I: Attachment. New York, NY: Basic Books.

Boyce, P. & Parker, G. (1989). Development of a scale to measure interpersonal sensitivity. Australian and New Zealand Journal of Psychiatry, 23, 341-351.

Briere, J., & Rickards, S. (2007). Self-awareness, affect regulation, and relatedness: Differential sequels of childhood versus adult victimization experiences. Journal of Nerv and Mental Disease, 195, 497-503.

Butovskaya, M., Boyko, E., Selverova, N. and Ermakova, I. (2005). The hormonal basis of reconciliation in humans. Journal of Physiological Anthropology and Applied Human Science, 24(4): 333-337.

Cords, M. & Killen, M. (1998). Conflict resolution in human and nonhuman primates. In J. Langer & M. Killen (Eds.). Piaget, evolution, and development (pp. 193-218). Mahwah, NJ.:Erlbaum Associates.

Costa, P. & McCrae, R. (1980). Influence of extraversion and neuroticism on subjective well-being: Happy and unhappy people. Journal of Personality and Social Psychology, 38, 668-678.

Couch, L. Jones, W. & Moore, D. (1999). Buffering the effects of betrayal: The role of apology, forgiveness, and commitment. In J. M. Adams & W. H. Jones (Eds.), Handbook of interpersonal commitment and relationship stability (pp. 451-469). New York, NY.: Kluwer Academic/Plenum Publishers.

Davenport, D. (1991). The functions of anger and forgiveness: Guidelines for psychotherapy with victims. Psychotherapy, 28, 140-144.

Girard, M. & Mullet, E. (1997). Propensity to forgive in adolescents, young adults, older adults, and elderly people. Journal of Adult Development, 4, 209-220.

Gobin, R. (2012). Partner preferences among survivors of betrayal trauma. J Trauma Dissociation, 13(2):152-74.

Goldman-Rakic, P. (1995). Architecture of the prefrontal cortex and the central executive. Ann. N.Y. Acad. Sci. 769, 71-83.

Gordon, K.C. & Baucom, D.H. (1998). Understanding betrayals in marriage: a synthesized model of forgiveness. Fam Process, 37(4), 425-49.

Kennell, J., Klaus, M., McGrath, S., Robertson, S. & Hinkley, C. (1991). Continuous emotional support during labor in U.S. hospital: A randomized control trial. Journal of the American Medical Association, 265, 2197-2201.

Lane, E.J., Lating, J.M., Lowry, J.L. & Martino, T.P. (2010). Differences in compassion fatigue, symptoms of posttraumatic stress disorder and relationship satisfaction, including sexual desire and functioning, between male and female detectives who investigate sexual offenses against children: a pilot study. Int J Emerg Ment Health., 12(4), 257-66.

Linden, W., Earl, T., Gerin, W. & Christenfeld, N. (1997). Physiological stress reactivity and recovery: Conceptual siblings separated at birth. J. Psychosom. Res. 42:117-135.

Lipton, B. (2005). The biology of belief: Unleashing the power of consciousness, matter, and miracles. New York, NY.: Hay House Publications.

Madones, C. (1991). Strategic family therapy (pp. 396-416). In A.S. Gurman and D.P. Kniskern (eds.), Handbook of family therapy (Vol. II). New York, NY: Brunner/Mazel.

McCann, I., Sakheim, D., & Abrahamson, D. (1988). Trauma and victimization: A model of psychological adaptation. The Counseling Psychologist, 16, 531-594.

Moritz, S., Kelly, M.T., Xu TJ, Toews, J., Rickhi, B. (2011). A spirituality teaching program for depression: qualitative findings on cognitive and emotional change. Complementary Therapies in Medicine, 19(4), 201-7.

Najavits, L. (2003). Seeking safety: a new psychotherapy for posttraumatic stress disorder and substance abuse disorder. In: Ouimette, P. & Brown, P. (Eds.) Trauma and substance abuse. Washington DC.: APA, pp. 147-169.

Ogrodniczuk, J., Piper, W., Joyce, A., McCallum, M., Rosie, J. (2003). NEO-five factor personality traits as predictors of response to two forms of group psychotherapy. Internal Journal of Group Psychotherapy, 53, 417-442.

Ohbuchi, K, Kameda, M. & Agarie, N. (1989). Aplogy as aggression control: Its role in mediating appraisal of and response to harm. J. Pers. Soc. Psychol. 56: 219-227.

Pukall, C. et al. (2007). Effectiveness of hypnosis for the treatment of vulvar vestibulitis syndrome: a preliminary investigation. J. Sex. Med., 4:417-425.

Shapiro, F. (2001). Eye movement desensitization and reprocessing: Basic principles, protocols and procedures, 2nd ed. New York, NY.: Guilford.

Seigel, D. (2010). Mindsight: The new science of personal transformation. New York, NY.: Random House.

Singer, J. & Salovey, P. (1988). Mood and memory: Evaluating the network theory of affect. Clinical Psychology Review, 8, 211-251.

Singer, T. (1996). The neuronal basis and ontogeny of empathy and mind reading: Review of literature and implications for future research. Neuroscience and Biobehavioral Reviews, 30, 855-863.

Steinberger, A., Payne, J, & Kensinger, E. (2011). The effect of cognitive reappraisal on the emotional memory trade-off. Cognition & Emotion, 25(7).

Chapter 16: Forgiveness-the Last Piece of the Puzzle

Aschleman, K. A. (1996). Forgiveness as a resiliency factor in divorced or permanently separated families. Unpublished master's thesis. Madison, WI: University of Wisconsin.

Bono, G., McCullough, M. E. & Root, L. (2006). Forgiveness and well-being. Coral Gables, FL.: University of Miami.

Bono, G., McCullough, M. E. & Root, L. (2007). Forgiveness, feeling connected to others, and well-being: Two longitudinal studies. Personality and Social Psychology Bulletin, 20(1): 1-14.

Boon, S. D. & Sulsky, L. M. (1997). Attributions of blame and forgiveness in romantic relationships: A policy-capturing study. Journal of Social Behavior and Personality, 12, 19-44.

Brown, R. (2003). Measuring individual differences in the tendency to forgive: Construct validity and links with depression. Personality and Social Psychology Bulletin, 29, 759-771.

Casarjian, R. (1992). Forgiveness: A bold choice for a peaceful heart. New York, NY.: Bantam.

DeShea, L, Tzou, J., Kang, S. & Matsuyuki, M. (2006). Trait forgiveness II: Spiritual vs religious college students and the five factor model of personality. Presented at the Annual Conference of the Society for Personality and Social Psychology, Palm, Springs, CA.

De Waal, F. (2003). The age of empathy: Nature's lessons for a kinder society. New York, NY.: Three Rivers Press.

Enright, R. D. (2001). Forgiveness is a choice; A step by step process for resolving anger and restoring hope. Washington, D.C., American Psychological Association.

Enright, R. D. (2000). Helping clients forgive; An emperical guide for resolving anger and restoring hope. Washington, D.C., American Psychological Association.

Enright, R. D., & North, J. (1998). Exploring forgiveness. Madison, Wisconsin, The University of Wisconsin Press.

Enright, R. D. and the Human Development Study Group, (1991). The moral development of forgiveness (pp. 123-152). In W. Kurtines & J. Gewirtz (eds.), Handbook of moral behavior and development, Hillsdale, NR: Lawrence Erlbaum Associates.

Exline, J. J., Baumeister, R. F., Bushman, B., Campbell, W. & Finkel, J. (2004). Too proud to let go: Narcissistic entitlement as a barrier to forgiveness. Journal of Personality and Social Psychology, 87, 894 912.

Exline, J. J., Worthington, E. L., Jr., Hill, P. C., & McCullough, M. E. (2003). Forgiveness and justice: A research agenda for social and personality psychology. Personality and Social Psychology Review, 7, 337-348.

Fincham, F. (2000). The kiss of the porcupines: From attributing responsibility to forgiving. Personal Relationships, 7, 1-23.

Friedberg, J.P., Suchday, S. & Shelov, D.V. (2007). The impact of forgiveness on cardiovascular reactivity and recovery. Int J Psychophysiol., 65(2), 87-94.

Hoyt, W. T. & McCullough, M. E. (2005). Issues in the multimodal measurement of forgiveness. In E.L. Worthington Jr. (Ed.), Handbook of Forgiveness (pp. 109-123). New York, NY.: Brunner-Routledge.

Karremans, J, Van Lange, P., Ouwerkerk, J, & Kluwer, E. (2003). When forgiving enhances psychological well-being: The role of interpersonal commitment. Journal of Personality and Social Psychology, 84, 1011-1026.

Karremans, J.& Van Lange, P. (2004). Back to caring after being hurt: The role of forgiveness. European Journal of Social Psychology, 34, 207-227.

Lawler-Row, K.A., Karremans, J.C., Scott, C., Edlis-Matityahou, M., & Edwards, L. (2008). Forgiveness, physiological reactivity and health: the role of anger. Int J Psychophysiol, 68(1),51-8.

Lawler K.A., Younger J.W., Piferi R.L., Jobe R.L., Edmondson K.A. & Jones W.H. (2005). The unique effects of forgiveness on health: an exploration of pathways. Journal of Behavioral Med., 28(2), 157-67.

Lawler K.A. et al. (2003). A change of heart: cardiovascular correlates of forgiveness in response to interpersonal conflict. J Behav Med., 26(5), 373-93.

Levenson MR, Aldwin CM, & Yancura L. (2006). Positive emotional change: mediating effects of forgiveness and spirituality. Explore, 2(6), 498-508.

Luskin, F. (2002). Forgive for good; A proven prescription for health and happiness. New York, NY.: Harper Collins Publishers.

McCullough, M. E., Luna, L. R., Berry, J. W., Tabak, B. A., & Bono, G. (2010). On the form and function of forgiving: Modeling the time-forgiveness relationship and testing the valuable relationships hypothesis. Emotion, 10, 358-376.

McCullough, M. E. et al. (2009). Forgiveness. In S.J. Lopez (Ed.), Handbook of positive psychology (2nd ed.), pp. 427-435. New York, NY.: Oxford.

McCullough, M.E. (2008). Beyond revenge: The evolution of the forgiveness instinct. San Francisco, CA.: Jossey-Bass.

McCullough, M. E., Bono, G., & Root, L. M. (2007). Rumination, emotion, and forgiveness: Three longitudinal studies. Journal of Personality and Social Psychology, 92, 490-505.

McCullough, M. E., Root, L. M., & Cohen, A. D. (2006). Writing about the benefits of an interpersonal transgression facilitates forgiveness. Journal of Consulting and Clinical Psychology, 74, 887-897.

McCullough, M. E., Fincham, F. D., & Tsang, J. (2003). Forgiveness, forbearance, and time: The temporal unfolding of transgression-related interpersonal motivations. Journal of Personality and Social Psychology, 84, 540-557.

McCullough, M. E. (2001). Forgiveness: who does it and how do they do it? Current Directions in Psychological Science, 10, 194-197.

McCullough, M. E. (2000). Forgiveness as human strength: Theory, measurement, and links to well-being. Journal of Social and Clinical Psychology, 19, 43-55.

McCullough, M. E. (2000) Forgiveness: Theory, research, and practice. New York, NY., Guilford Press.

McCullough, M. E., & Worthington, E. L., Jr. (1999). Religion and the forgiving personality. Journal of Personality, 67, 1141-1164.

McCullough, M. E. et al. (1998). Interpersonal forgiving in close relationships: II. Theoretical elaboration and measurement. Journal of Personality and Social Psychology, 75, 1586-1603.

McCullough, M. E., Worthington, E. L., Jr., & Rachal, K. C. (1997). Interpersonal forgiving in close relationships. Journal of Personality and Social Psychology, 77, p. 218.

McCullough, M. E., Sandange, S. J., & Worthington, E. L. (1997). To forgive is human; How to put your past in the past. Downers Grove, IL., Intervarsity Press.

McFarland, M.J., Smith, C.A., Toussaint, L. & Thomas, P.A. (2012). Forgiveness of others and health: do race and neighborhood matter? J Gerontol B Psychol Sci Soc Sci., 67(1), 66-75.

Murphy, J. (1982). Forgiveness and resentment. Midwest Studies in Philosophy, 7, 503-516.

Newberg, A., d'Aquili, E., Newberg, S. & deMarici, V. (2000). The neuropsychological correlates of forgiveness. In: Forgiveness: Theory, Research, and Practice by McCullough, M., Pargament, K. and Thoresen, C. (Eds.). New York, NY.: Guilford.

Pingleton, J. (1989). The role and function of forgiveness in the psychotherapeutic process. Journal of Psychology and Theology, 17, 27-35.

Rosenak, C. & Harnden, G. (1992). Forgiveness in the psychotherapeutic process: Clinical applications. Journal of Psychology and Christianity, 11, 188-197.

Rowe, J. et al. (1989). The psychology of forgiving another: A dialogal research approach (pp. 233-244). In R.S. Valle & S. Halling (eds.), Existential-phenomenological perspectives in psychology: Exploring the breadth of human experience. New York, NY: Plenum Press.

Smedes, L. (1996). The art of forgiving: When you need to forgive and don't know how. New York, NY.: Ballantine.

Smedes, L. (1984). Forgive and forget: Healing the hurts we don't deserve. New York, NY: Harper & Row.

Tabak, B. A., McCullough, M. E., Root, L. M., Bono, G., & Berry, J. W. (2011). Conciliatory gestures facilitate forgiveness and feelings of friendship by making transgressors seem more agreeable. Journal of Personality (in press).

Thompson, L. et al. (2005). Dispositional forgiveness of self, others, and situations. Journal of Personality, 73, 313-359.

Tomm, K. (1999) Enabling forgiveness and reconciliation in family therapy. Retrieved from: http://www.familytherapy.org/documents/enabling_forgivess_ktom.pdf

Tsang, J., McCullough, M. E., & Fincham, F. D. (2006). The longitudinal association between forgiveness and relationship closeness and commitment. Journal of Social and Clinical Psychology, 25, 448-472.

Weinar, B., Graham, S., Peter, O., & Zmuidinas, M. (1991). Public confession and forgiveness. Journal of Personality, 59, 281-314.

Whited, M.C., Wheat, A.L. & Larkin, K.T. (2010). The influence of forgiveness and apology on cardiovascular reactivity and recovery in response to mental stress. J Behav Med., 33(4), 293-304.

Witvliet, C., Ludwig, T., & Vander Laan, K. (2001). Granting forgiveness or harboring grudges: Implications for emotion, physiology, and health. Psychological Science, 12, 117-123.

Worthington, E.L. & Scherer, M. (2004). Forgiveness as an emotion-focused coping strategy that can reduce health risks and promote health resilience: Theory, review, and hypotheses. Psychology and Health, 19, 385-405.

Worthington, E. L. (2003). Forgiving and reconciling: Bridges to wholeness and hope. Madison, WI.: Inter varsity Press.

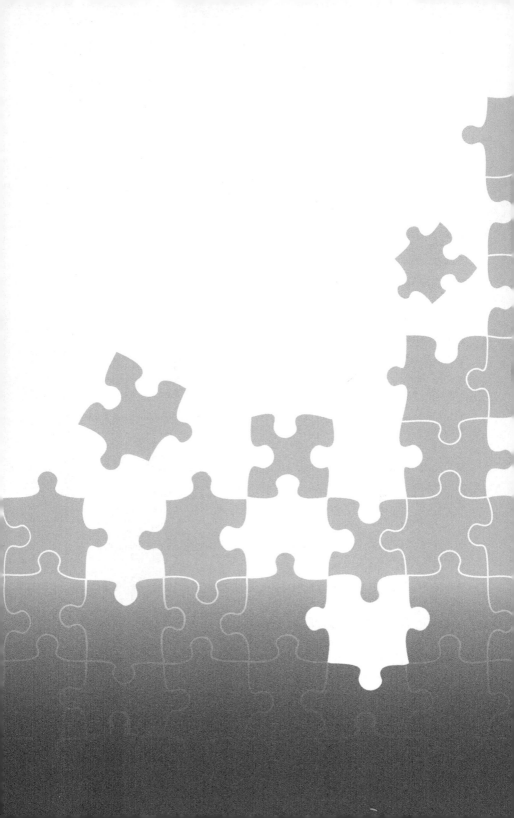